**ENERGY**
THE SPARK OF LIFE &
UNIVERSAL GODDESS

Other books by Swami Muktibodhananda Saraswati,

*Swara Yoga the Tantric Science of Brain Breathing*

*Commentaries on Hatha Yoga Pradipika,*
*the Light on Hatha Yoga.*

Both published by the Bihar School of Yoga.

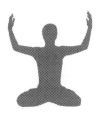

# ENERGY
## THE SPARK OF LIFE &
# UNIVERSAL GODDESS
### A BOOK ABOUT YOGA AND
### PERSONAL GROWTH FOR MEN AND WOMEN

Swami Muktibodhananda Saraswati

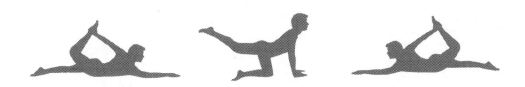

Order this book online at www.trafford.com
or email orders@trafford.com

Most Trafford titles are also available at major online book retailers.

Print information available on the last page.

ISBN: 978-1-4120-6930-4 (sc)
ISBN: 978-1-4251-9536-6 (e)

*Trafford rev. 07/20/2018*

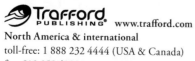
www.trafford.com
North America & international
toll-free: 1 888 232 4444 (USA & Canada)
fax: 812 355 4082

# TABLE OF CONTENTS

Acknowledgements . . . . . . . . . . . . . . . . . . . . . . . . . . . 2

Introduction . . . . . . . . . . . . . . . . . . . . . . . . . . . 3

Pronunciation of Sanskrit vowels and consonants . . . . . . . 4

A Meditation . . . . . . . . . . . . . . . . . . . . . . . . . 6

Chapter One     The Universal Goddess: Energy . . . . . . . . . . . . 7

Chapter Two     Healthy Attitudes . . . . . . . . . . . . . . . . . . . 21

Chapter Three     Yoga Cleansing Practices . . . . . . . . . . . . . . . 27

Chapter Four     Body Stabilization: Asana . . . . . . . . . . . . . . 31

Chapter Five     Breath Utilisation: Pranayama . . . . . . . . . . . . 67

Chapter Six     Muscle Squeezing: Bandha . . . . . . . . . . . . . . 75

Chapter Seven     Energy Gestures: Mudra . . . . . . . . . . . . . . . 79

Chapter Eight     Mind Absorption: Meditation . . . . . . . . . . . . 89

Chapter Nine     Food and Health Tips . . . . . . . . . . . . . . . . 101

Chapter Ten     Relationships and Family . . . . . . . . . . . . . . 111

Further Reading . . . . . . . . . . . . . . . . . . . . . . . 116

About the Author . . . . . . . . . . . . . . . . . . . . . . 117

## ACKNOWLEDGEMENTS

Special acknowledgements go to my mother,
Virginia Hayward-Nash (Nityamuktananda),
for enabling me to pursue yoga,
and for her positive input towards publishing this book;
to my teacher, mentor and Guru,
Paramahansa Swami Satyananda Saraswati;
to Swami Sambuddhananda for the lovely painting used on the covers of the book;
to Sakshi Winning for her constructive comments;
to Joss Guin, a dedicated sadhaka aspirant, who was my yoga model;
to Suzi Tooke for her editing;
to my Uncle and Aunt,
Rod and Liz Nash and their design student intern Anil Singh
(Nash & Nash Ltd., Canada), for their design and artwork that helped turn the
manuscript into a user-friendly book;
to all the people I have taught and for their input in my life as a teacher;
and to you for being interested in your own self development.

# INTRODUCTION

I remember as a child telling my mother that I would write a book when I was 40. Actually my first two books were written in my twenties when I was inspired to delve into the deeper aspects of yoga and advanced practices. But after teaching many aspects of yoga in Australia over the last 20 years I found a need for a different style of yoga book that integrated the profound knowledge of yoga with a Western lifestyle.

There are plenty of yoga books these days that can instruct you in the correct art of yoga posture or books that discuss yoga philosophy. So how do you integrate this knowledge with your day-to-day life? Is your spiritual life separate from your worldly life? I have noticed that many people have a conflict between their understanding of what is spiritual and what is physical. If you have this inner conflict you need to find a method that enables you to experience your mind, body and soul/consciousness as a complete being. When you realize the expression of soul/consciousness in every cell of your body, you can experience true joyousness. Personally I have found yoga can assist with this realization. Yoga does not interfere with your religious beliefs. As you do the practices you will have your own inner realizations about your self, the other people in your life, and your environment. This book is the product of my heart-felt need for all yoga teachers and aspirants to imbibe the essence of yoga, and its practical application in life. It is the culmination of my past 30 years of teaching in the east and west, and is a unique book incorporating the fundamentals of yoga with a western understanding.

May your heart sing and inner vision be clear.

(Muktibodha)

## PRONUNCIATION OF SANSKRIT VOWELS AND CONSONANTS

The traditions of *tantra* and *yoga* were originally recorded in the ancient language of Sanskrit. Sanskrit is written in the *deva nagari* script. Unlike English, sanskrit is phonetic. When reading a translation of Sanskrit in roman script, which is how we read English, there can be some confusion of the exact pronunciation.

Sanskrit is an unadulterated language. It was realized in deep states of meditation. Each sound has an influence on your mind and body. It is, therefore, useful to repeat the sounds and understand the concepts. Each sound is an aspect of the Universal Goddess and manifests within everything animate and inanimate. By repeating these sounds, we trace our journey back to the Universal Goddess.

To assist you with correct pronunciation of the terminology used, here is a list defining each sound. The vowels with a line underneath indicate a long vowel sound. Consonants followed by an 'h' are aspirated. For example, in Sanskrit there is no 'th' as in 'the'; the sound is 't' with an aspiration from the throat following it. Some sounds in Sanskrit are not used in English and it can take a little practice to become familiar with these new sounds.

## Vowel pronunciation

अ    **a**    as in s*u*n
आ    **a̱**    as in f*a*ster
इ    **i**    as in *i*t
ई    **e̱**    as in *ee*l
उ    **u**    as in b*u*ll
ऊ    **u̱**    as in sch*oo*l
ऋ    **ri**    rolled r sound followed by i
ॠ    **ṟi**    rolled r sound followed by ee
ऌ    **lri** l +rolled r followed by I
ॡ    **lṟi** l +rolled r followed by ee
ए    **e**    as in *ai*d
ऐ    **ai**    as in b*ye*
ओ    **o**    as in j*o*g
औ    **au** as in h*ow*

## Consonant pronunciation

In the Sanskrit alphabet, consonants are automatically pronounced with an 'a' sound (s*u*n) following the consonant, e.g. ka, unless otherwise indicated. The following list describes each consonant without the 'a' sound and, therefore, to be technically correct each Sanskrit consonant has a small line beneath it, e.g. क् k.

क्    **k**    as in jun*k*
ख्    **kh**    k followed by an aspirated h, as in blac*kh*ead
ग्    **g**    as in ba*g*
घ्    **gh**    g followed by an aspirated h, as in do*gh*ouse
ङ्    **n**    nasal sounding n, as in hu*n*k

| | | | | | | |
|---|---|---|---|---|---|---|
| चू | ch | as in *ch*ew | | श् | sh | as in *sh*ut |
| छ् | chh | ch followed by an aspirated h, as in lun*ch h*abit | | ष् | s | half way between sh and s |
| ज् | j | as in *j*ug | | स् | s | as in *s*at |
| झ् | jh | j followed by aspirated h, as in ca*ge h*im | | ह् | h | as in *h*ungry |
| ञ् | ny | as in o*ni*on | | क्ष् | ksh | as in boo*k sh*op |
| ट् | t | pronounced on the palate, i.e. palatal t, as in *t*ea | | ज्ञ् | gy | as in sa*ng y*ou |
| ठ् | th | palatal t followed by aspirated h, as in fi*t h*im | | | | |
| ड् | d | palatal d as in *d*og | | | | |
| ढ् | dh | palatal d followed by aspirated h, as in ba*d h*and | | | | |
| ण् | rn | as in bu*rn* | | | | |
| त् | t | dental t sound, pronounced behind the front teeth | | | | |
| थ् | th | dental t sound followed by an aspirated h | | | | |
| द् | d | dental d sound, pronounced behind the front teeth | | | | |
| ध् | dh | dental d sound followed by an aspirated h | | | | |
| न् | n | as in no*n* | | | | |
| प् | p | as in jum*p* | | | | |
| फ् | ph | p followed by an aspirated h, as in tra*p h*im | | | | |
| ब् | b | as in ja*b* | | | | |
| भ् | bh | b followed by an aspirated h, as in jo*b h*unt | | | | |
| म् | m | as in *m*um | | | | |
| य् | y | as in *y*et | | | | |
| र् | r | as in bea*r* | | | | |
| ल् | l | as in wil*l* | | | | |
| व् | v | as in *v*ase | | | | |

*Aum bh<u>u</u>r bhuva sw<u>a</u>ha*
*Tat savitur varenyam*
*Bhargo devasya dh<u>i</u>mahi*
*Dhiyo yo naha prachoday<u>a</u>t*

*(G<u>a</u>yatr<u>i</u> Mantra)*


We meditate upon
the radiant divine light
of that adorable sun of spiritual consciousness.
May it awaken
our intuitional consciousness.

# CHAPTER ONE

# The Universal Goddess: Energy

*I am hurt.*
*I am angry.*
*I'm happy, I'm sad.*
*I'm in pain, I feel sorrow and grief.*
*I'm ecstatic, elated and over the moon.*
*I'm quiet and peaceful and still.*
*What am I?*

(Muktibodha)

## The Spark Of Life

As this book has caught your attention you must be seeking deeper expression in your life, consciously or unconsciously. Perhaps you feel hungry at some inner level and can't quite pinpoint what you need. Maybe life has thrown you into difficult circumstances and you are trying to make sense of it all. Or you could be in a situation where you feel unsupported in your life and wonder where to turn. Life has a tendency to put you in a situation where you can grow. These situations are often difficult because it is not easy to change old habits or adjust to new challenges or see yourself objectively. However, the right answers for you will be there when you search for them. And so this book can be a stepping-stone towards fulfilling your personal goals.

In order to understand yourself and your world you need to realize that life is not only a material manifestation. The physical world and your expression in it are both an important part of your experience but not your total existence. There are subtler aspects of which to become aware. Whether you are atheist, agnostic or theist you need fulfillment on all levels from the physical, to mental, emotional and intuitional layers. A theist will search for meaning in life through a personal understanding of God, the scientist searches for meaning through the intellect and scientific evidence or theories of quantum physics/mechanics, an atheist will search for meaning through evidence in the material world and a *yogi* or *tantrik* comprehends this directly through meditation. Perhaps you have perceived it through your own inner knowing or inner faith or intuitive experience. If you haven't found it yet then you may even doubt your ability to ever find the true meaning. However, after reading this book and following the practices you will have a better understanding of yourself and your personal process of inner fulfillment.

First it is essential to realize that you are a conglomerate of physical and energetic components that give you life. While you can see and feel your physical body there are subtler forces that endow you with life. The standard model of cosmology today describes that the visible universe contains approximately 5% ordinary matter, 25% dark matter and 70% dark energy. The true nature of this dark matter and energy is a big mystery in cosmology. *Tantra* and *yoga* describe this dark energy and matter as the primordial goddess known as **prana**, **shakti** or **prakriti**. This goddess is the vehicle of universal consciousness known as **chit**, **shiva** or **purusha**.

According to *tantra* and *yoga* philosophy the universal goddess energy and consciousness coexist as polarities in both the manifest and unmanifest world. And so it is in within each individual. Your consciousness is a force more subtle than your brain and mind or anything you may perceive in the physical realm. The view of modern medicine is that consciousness is a product of the brain, that a baby is born and thereby endowed with consciousness. *Yoga* describes that form of consciousness as mental consciousness. Science also explains consciousness as the subtle form of energy, and energy the subtle form of matter, just as gas is the subtle manifestation of liquid and solid. The subtle point or seed of consciousness within you is the reflection of the universal consciousness. Some call this the Spark of Life. Because it is a form of energy, the feminine principle, it is called the goddess. The goddess manifests consciousness and life force in the material world.

Every human being is made of the same atoms as stars. That which endows you with individual consciousness is the goddess consciousness. When you came into the world your inner goddess was possibly dormant waiting to be nurtured to full maturity. Maybe your goddess had already manifested but was later sadly suppressed, being forced to retreat deep within. Set your goddess free. Your goddess is not subject to duality, time or space, night or day, male or female, opposites or polarities, health or disease, pain or pleasure. The goddess is always there for you, always ready with endless love and light irrespective of who and how you are in the world. The goddess is nameless, give whatever name suits you it does not change the goddess. What does change is your perception, experience and your relationship to yourself. To experience this goddessness within you, first understand your inner makeup.

## What constitutes mind

An individual mind is known as an inner organ *antah karana*. It has many facets. *Ahamkara*, the external personality *and ego* is one aspect of the mind. You were born with an immature ego which developed according to your circumstances, parents, social and religious conditioning. These are the factors that mould your personality. Another aspect is the mental content *chitta* that includes the subconscious and unconscious layers. It consists of your ability to cognize, concentrate and remember. It is the store of all your memories, including unconscious memories inherited from your ancestral gene pool. The next aspect of mind is intellect *buddhi*, i.e. your ability to analyze, assess, evaluate and to be practical. Sometimes mind as a whole is referred to as *manas* and mental energy as *manas shakti*. To be very specific, *manas* is the aspect of your mind which constantly chatters. The four mental aspects operate in conjunction with your *indriya* senses of smell, taste, sight, touch or sensation and hearing. The subtlest aspect of your mind is intuition, *pragya*. Your intuition knows without external stimuli, without your senses or any other part of your mind. It is the closest aspect of you to goddessness. Intuition is the first to perceive Self and

allows goddessness to be felt by every layer of your being.

Generally people only use one tenth of their total brain capacity. So what is the remaining nine tenths capable of? As you practice *yoga* you may find you are capable of achieving much more than at present. Some of the essential practices are elucidated here in this book.

## What constitutes the body

Modern science can explicitly explain to you the chemical and anatomical structure of your physical body. However, these chemical components can only manifest because of a decrease in the frequency of the inherent consciousness. Now it is your endeavor to realize this process by retracing your goddess' descent into your body.

*Yoga* and *tantra* describe human existence to consist of five layers. Each layer, known as *kosha*, is interactive with the other. They do not function independently; they are symbiotic.

The first and most subtle layer is comprised of ecstasy or bliss *ananda-maya kosha*; next is the intuitive layer *vigyana-maya kosha*; third layer is the mental covering *mano-maya kosha* consisting of the four aspects of mind discussed previously. The fourth layer consists of subtle *pranic* energy *prana-maya kosha* and the fifth layer is made of food *anna-maya kosha*. According to the authorities on *yoga* and *tantra*, *pranamaya kosha* consists of 72,000 *nadi* energy pathways, 10 **vayu** energy currents, and seven main **chakra** energy/consciousness centers. The fifth and last layer **anna-maya kosha** is made of the food you eat. When there is an imbalance in one of the *kosha* layers the other *kosha* layers are also affected. Therefore, to heal a problem it is important to employ methods that assist the different layers. By practising specific techniques of *yoga* and *tantra*, that influ-

ence your *pranamaya kosha*, you can directly affect your experience of goddessness in the *anandamaya kosha*

Your body is also made up of five **tattwa** elemental components:

*Prithvi tattwa* **earth element:** the force which creates cohesiveness and binds all the components of the body together, the infrastructure, skeletal system, marrow and blood.

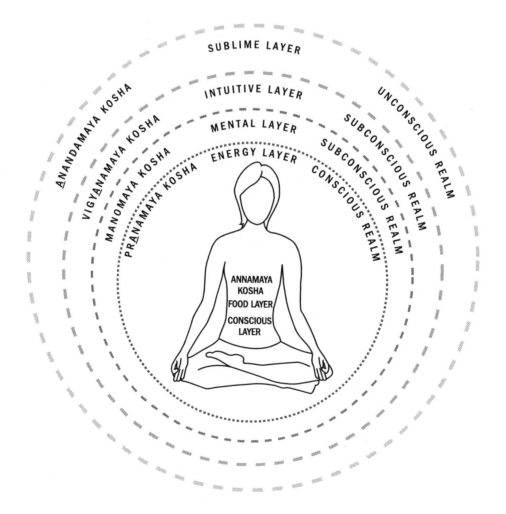

*Apas tattwa* **water element:**
body fluids.

*Agni tattwa* **fire element:**
the power of the digestive fire and ability to sleep.

*Vayu tattwa* **air element:**
muscle expansion and contraction, emotions and passions.

*Akasha tattwa* **ether element:**
the force which is space giving and which separates each different part and organ.

There are also subtle energy currents that motivate various areas of the body known as *prana vayu*. *Vayu* literally means flow of air. *Prana vayu* is a general term referring to five main currents of subtle energy that flow in different directions through your body:

*Apana vayu:*
the force of expulsion below the navel which enables a bowel motion and birthing.

*Prana vayu:*
the upward moving force above the navel which enables breathing.

*Samana vayu:*
the middle force, which equalizes *apana* and *prana vayu*.

*Udana vayu:*
the force functioning the throat, speech and facial expression.

*Vyana vayu:*
the force which circulates energy throughout the body regulating circulation and the exchange of nutrients.

There are also five subsidiary *prana vayu*, **upaprana,** complementing the above mentioned functions, causing blinking, hunger, thirst, sneezing, coughing and the remaining cellular life after death.

Goddess consciousness and energy are also conducted along three specific channels in your body known as **nadi** energy flows. The word *nadi* literally means river. These three flows have a positive or negative or neutral charge. The subtle energy powering your mind is considered to be the negative charge called **manas shakti** and travels through the pathway known as **ida nadi.**

The subtle energy powering your body is considered to be a positive charge called **prana shakti** and flows through the pathway known as **pingala nadi.** The neutral energy is divine and flows through the central axis of your spine known as **sushumna nadi.**

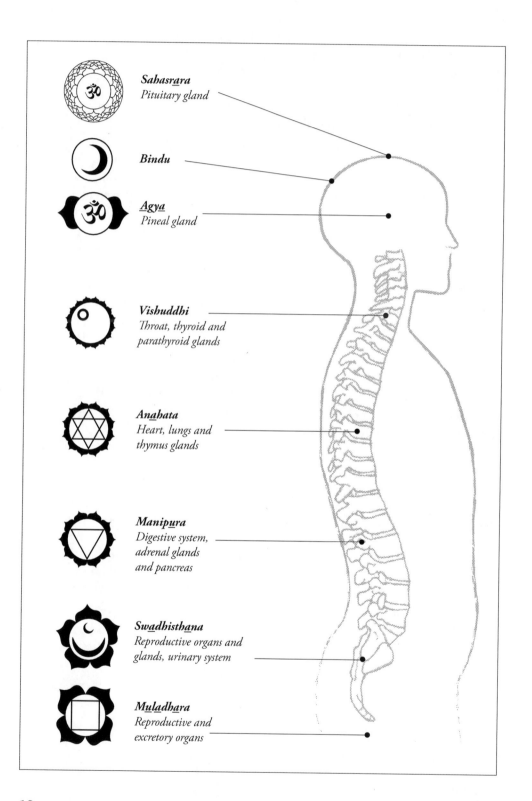

**Sahasrara**
*Pituitary gland*

**Bindu**

**Agya**
*Pineal gland*

**Vishuddhi**
*Throat, thyroid and parathyroid glands*

**Anahata**
*Heart, lungs and thymus glands*

**Manipura**
*Digestive system, adrenal glands and pancreas*

**Swadhisthana**
*Reproductive organs and glands, urinary system*

**Muladhara**
*Reproductive and excretory organs*

## Chakra vortices

Within your body the subtle energy pathways of *ida* and *pingala* meet along the axis of *sushumna*. These meeting points are known as **chakra** junctions. Each *chakra* junction is a swirling mass of vital *prana* and mental *manasik* energy. Seven *chakra* vortices located along the central axis of your body are most significant. While the *chakra* system is perceived within the *pranamaya* layer, each *chakra* is a trigger point and portal between the physical, mental and psychic realms. Each *chakra* has an influence over associated organs and senses, resulting in certain physiological and psychological experiences. Likewise, the action of a specific organ or gland can influence a *chakra* and even your thoughts can affect a specific *chakra*.

There are five main *chakra* vortices located in proximity to the spinal column and nerve plexus. At the south polar base of your spine is the slowest vibrating *chakra* and at the north polar top of the spinal axis and crown of the head is the fastest vibrating *chakra* vortex. *Chakra* vortices are often depicted as flowers, usually the lotus because of its spiritual significance.

The lotus's roots go deep into the mud, the stem grows straight up through the water and the flower blooms upward facing the sky, just like the consciousness moving from the physical earth plain and on towards heaven, the subtler realms and beyond. *Muladhara* and *sahasrara's* orientations face downwards because they are gateways between different realms while the other *chakra* centres face upwards. Below *muladhara* are the animal, insect and vegetable kingdoms and above *sahasrara* are the divine realms.

According to *yoga* and *tantra* the *chakra* vortices are called:

*Muladhara:* the 'base support': behind the female cervix or within the male perineum.

*Swadhisthana:* 'one's own dwelling place': at the sacral spine parallel to the pubic bone.

*Manipura:* the 'city of jewels': in the thoracic spine above the navel.

*Anahata:* the 'unstruck sound': in the thoracic spine level with the sternum.

*Vishuddhi:* the 'great purifier': in the cervical spine level with the Adams apple.

*Agya:* 'command': towards mid brain level with the eyebrow centre.

*Sahasrara:* 'one thousand (petals)': crown of head

*Bindu:* the 'single point': is a psychic centre located at the top back portion of the head where *Hare Krishna* devotees leave a tuft of hair. It works in conjunction with *agya* and *sahasrara*.

*Copy continues on page 16*

*This chart describes the various manifestations of the Goddess within.*

| Chakras: | MULADHARA | SWADHISTHANA | MANIPURA |
|---|---|---|---|
| Physical organs & glands | coccygeal plexus cervix perineal floor bowels | sacral plexus, urogenital system reproductive glands intestines | solar plexus digestive system adrenal glands |
| Positive & negative attributes | survival, self preservation, tribal, animal instincts, trust, nationalism, patriotism, grounding, steadfastness, prosperity, resentment, deep seated fear, undisciplined, dullness, slothfulness, monotony, materialism, hoarding | addictions, fear, setting or lack of boundaries, lacking self worth, self gratification, sexuality & power, desire to feel & want, guilt, obsessiveness, | ability or inability to exert will power, purpose, domination, subordination, high or low self esteem, self definition, vitality, anger, joy, laughter, spontaneity, responsibility, finances, aggrandizing, shame, blaming, |
| Individual expression | I have | I want, I desire | I can, I will |
| Physical ailments | languor & laziness, over or under weight, constipation, hemorrhoids, coccygeal problems | reproductive, bladder or urinary & sacral & lumbar spine problems, frigidity, impotency | ulcers, diabetes hypoglycemia, chronic fatigue, lethargy, digestive disorders, thoracic spine problems |
| *Tattwa* element | earth *prithvi* | water *apas* | fire *agni* |
| Tattwa color | yellow | white | red |
| *Mantra* | *lam* | *vam* | *ram* |
| Tattwa function in body | skin, blood vessels, bone construction | all body fluids | appetite, thirst, sleep |
| *Gyanendriya* sense organ | nose | tongue | eyes |
| *Tanmatra* essence within the mind | smell | taste | sight |
| *Karmendriya* organ of action | anus | reproductive organs | feet/legs |

| ANAHATA | VISHUDDHI | AGYA | SAHASRARA |
|---|---|---|---|
| cardiac plexus, lungs, heart, thymus glands, immune system | cervical plexus, throat, tongue, ears, thyroid gland | pineal gland | pituitary gland |
| love, affection, compassion, good will, forgiveness, balance, self acceptance, empathy or lack of, social, fairness, clair sentience, grief, jealousy, bitterness, shyness, feelings of isolation & loneliness | absorb information & communicate, truth, listening & expressing, balance, excitement, clair audience, resonance, rhythm & timing, the need to create, inability and fear of speaking & listening, lying, denial, non-stop chatter, stuttering, pushing limits | clear vision & interpretation, self reflection, intuition, imagination, concentration, dreaming, psychic perception, clair voyance, delusions & illusions, denial, hallucinations, inability to concentrate or remember | intuitive knowing & understanding self knowledge, bliss, attachment, overly intellectual, confusion, addicted to spirituality, dissociation, |
| I love, I feel | I speak, I hear | I see, I perceive | I know, I understand |
| asthma, angina high BP, skin & nervous conditions thoracic spine problems | tonsil, thyroid & throat problems, cold/flu cervical spine problems | blindness, headaches, nightmares | confusion, mental depression, alienation |
| air *vayu* | ether *akasha* | mind *chitta* including intuition *pragya* | *chit* divine consciousness &, light *prakasha* |
| smokey blue | all colors | | |
| *yam* | *ham* | *aum* | *aum* |
| muscle expansion contraction | ether: emotions, passions | *chitta*: mental activity, telepathy clairvoyance, telekinesis, | *prakasha*: life essence |
| skin | ears | | |
| touch | hearing | | |
| hands/fingers | vocal cords | | |

The particular rate of vibration of each *chakra* vortex produces a specific color, sound and image.

*Muladhara* vibrates at a slow rate, creating a deep crimson color, the sound of **lam** (lum) and the image of a four petalled flower.

*Swadhisthana* produces a deep orange color, the sound **vam** (vum) and the form of a six petalled flower.

Manipura produces the image of a deep yellow 10 petalled flower and the sound of **ram** (rum).

*Anahata* produces the image of a pale blue 12 petalled flower and the sound **yam** (yum). Some people see anahata as being green. Attached to *anahata* is the wish fulfilling tree **kalpa vriksha** or **kalpa taru** which is green. Everyone's personal experience will vary and is valid. As *anahata* expresses unconditional love, it may even appear pink.

*Vishuddhi* produces the image of a 16 petalled purple flower and the sound **ham** (hum).

*Agya* is pure white and appears to have 2 petals, one on the right and the other on the left. The sound vibration manifesting here is that of *Aum*.

*Sahasrara* is also pure white light, it may appear to be all colors, the sound is *Aum* and it is said to have a thousand petals.

## Thousands of years ago

Thousands of years ago, various people in India experimented with different methods to achieve total integration of being. *Tantra* and *yoga* are the products of this experimentation. To give you some sort of time frame, archeological artifacts of *yoga asana* postures have been found in the Indus Valley dating back c3000 BC and linking it to the Indus-Saraswati civilization. Several *Hatha yoga* practices are also included in the system of health and spirituality of *Ayurvedic* medicine which some say dates back 10,000 years. There is also reference to *yoga* in other ancient *Vedic* books, which are many thousands of years old. So, suffice to say, *yoga* is very ancient and time tested.

The system of *Raja yoga* was initially formalized in written verse by *Patanjali* c500 BC. His work is known as the *Yoga Sutras*. In his *sutras*, *Patanjali* refers to the psychological and paranormal effects of specific *yoga* practices and meditation. The variety of physical *Hatha yoga* techniques were not written about until much later, between c12th and c15[th] AD and can be found in books such as *Goraksha Satarka*, *Gherand Samhita* and *Hatha Yoga Pradipika*. Nonetheless, *Hatha yoga* is a very ancient method employed by shamans and seekers to find physical, mental, emotional, psychic and spiritual well-being.

Both systems of *Hatha yoga* and *Raja yoga* utilise similar methods commencing with the physical body and conscious mind and culminating in transcendence of both. The original *Hatha yoga* texts mainly describe practices to harness the vital and mental energies, whereas *Patanjali's Yoga Sutras* deal with the psychological outcome of *yoga* practices and transcendence. Therefore, it is considered that *Raja yoga* is the culmination of *Hatha yoga*.

*Raja yoga* consists of eight stages or limbs. Firstly, it introduces ten personal guidelines; five **yama** restraints and five **niyama** observances. Gradually *yama* and *niyama* develop into spontaneous attitudes and virtues. When practising *Hatha yoga*, *yama* and *niyama* are adopted after cleaning the internal body through six cleansing techniques known as the **shat karma**. *Hatha yoga* also elucidates various postures, breathing, gestures and muscle contractions.

Just as you go to school and gain an intellectual education, by practising *Raja* or *Hatha yoga* regularly you train your intuitive mind to be sensitive to the subtler aspects of mind, psyche and energy.

*Asana* is the stage after body purification. An *asana* may either be a steady and comfortable sitting position that assists the process of meditation or a pose that enhances a particular bodily function. Practising various *asana* postures improves all the physiological systems, including muscle flexibility and strength, joint lubrication, regulation of endocrine gland secretioning and enhancing the digestive system. By practicing *asana* you generate physical and mental well-being.

*Pranayama* is the practice of breath control that unifies right and left brain hemisphere activities, improves functioning of the frontal lobes, stabilizes and strengthens the nervous system, as well as generating mental and physical energy. By breathing in different ways you can warm your body when the weather is cool, or cool your body when weather is hot. In terms of *Hatha yoga*, the ultimate goal of *pranayama* is reached when the process of breathing is spontaneously suspended. This is called **kevala kumbhaka** and the occurrence coincides with deep meditation.

*Mudra* is a physical gesture that promotes the flow of universal energy through your body and mind. Certain *mudra* gestures are practised to induce specific states of mental concentration.

*Bandha* is the practice of isolating and tensing specific muscle groups to harness physical and subtle energy flows. Bandha specifically energizes *muladhara*, *manipura* and *vishuddhi chakra* points. It draws together the two opposing flows of energy, i.e. *prana vayu* current which usually flows upward is drawn down to the navel and the downward flowing current of *apana vayu*, is pulled up to the navel.

*Pratyahara* is a state of being when you are able to witness yourself objectively. During the practice of *pratyahara* you sit or lie motionlessly observing the external stillness of your body while simultaneously being aware of each sense withdrawing from the external world. This may also occur while holding an *asana* posture. In the state of *pratyahara* the experience of your senses is directly within the mind itself. During sleep your senses withdraw from the external world, though you are unaware of it. In the dream state you experience directly through your mind itself. Without your senses interacting with an external object you can taste food, smell a fragrance or odor, see a scene, feel an object or hear sounds. Once you are able to be aware that you are dreaming while observing the dream itself, the process of dreaming can be developed into *pratyahara*.

*Dharana* occurs after *pratyahara*. You sit in a comfortable position that you know you can remain in for at least fifteen minutes. Keeping your eyes closed you focus your mind on the memory of an image, or you mentally repeat a *mantra* sound. Loosely translated *dharana* is concentration. In the actual state of *dharana* you are aware of yourself and the object you concentrating on. You are also aware of the state of witnessing, the eyes seeing, the stillness of your body, focus of your mind as well as distractions. The mind oscillates from focus to distraction during *dharana* and you witness all the mental tendencies and fluctuations while still focusing on the object of concentration. Dreaming can also be a process of *dharana* because your mind is already introverted and your body still.

In order for the dream state to become the state of *dharana* you will need to observe yourself dreaming and to control the subject of your dream; i.e. to decide what you are going to dream and see to that, though you will not have control of what unfolds you will be able only to choose the subject. By practising *dharana* you will become aware of the influence of your subconscious mind over your conscious mind, your decision-making and expression of your personality. Becoming aware of your subconscious tendencies enables you to make positive choices in life.

*Dhyana* is the state of consciousness after *dharana* when you are able to witness your mind absorbed in concentration of a particular subject while simultaneously witnessing that you are separate. The mind may be completely absorbed but it is the existence of your ego that creates the feeling of separateness. *Dhyana* is a spontaneous experience. *Pratyahara* and *dharana* are practised in order to induce *dhyana*. The state of deep unconscious sleep would become *dhyana* if you could be aware and witness yourself in that state. In this state your consciousness is absorbed into the collective unconscious and so it is not an easy task to maintain awareness in this state.

*Samadhi* is the progression of *dhyana*, gradually transcending the experience of "I"ness or ego. In deep sleep you do not know you exist, your mind has cut off from everything, but you are still alive and your body is there asleep on the bed.

In *samadhi* you are unconscious to the external world and body; however, you are aware of your existence and that you are experiencing your Self in some form that words cannot describe. The experience of "I"ness is not as you see yourself in the mirror but is just a trace of awareness that you do exist somewhere in a state of bliss unaffected by time or space. It is possible to have a tiny glimpse of this and, when the experience is over, life goes on as usual. There is a Zen saying, "Before enlightenment: chopping wood and carrying water. After enlightenment: chopping wood and carrying water." The world continues on in the same way after an experience of *samadhi*. However, your relationship with the world and people around you will definitely change.

Just as you go to school and gain an intellectual education, by regular practise of *Raja* or *Hatha yoga* you are sensitizing yourself to the subtler aspects of mind, psyche and energy. **You may not be able to practise every aspect of** *y**oga*,** so choose the techniques that suit your lifestyle.**

# CHAPTER 2

# Healthy Attitudes

*Atoms are not greedy,*
*The stars are not greedy*
*The earth is not greedy*
*Nature progresses within time and space.*
*But within the human mind breeds such a greed*
*that destroys and devours,*
*And annihilates all nature from time and space.*

(Muktibodha)

*Yoga* describes three states and stages of mind, matter and energy. Everything that exists evolves from an inert **tamasik** state/stage, to a dynamic and oscillating **rajasik** state/stage and onto the pure, balanced **sattvik** state/stage. The physical, *pranik* and mental bodies or layers are subject to these three **guna** states/stages. Humans are also evolving through these states/stages which means that your thought processes are going to change throughout your life and your attitudes will change accordingly.

A *tamasik* state of mind causes a negative approach to life. *The force of tamas is* exerting its influence when you are stuck in a rut. It is very difficult to change a

*tamasik* state and it requires an incredible thrust to move into the next *rajasik* phase of growth. *Rajasik* attitudes swing between negative and positive, between an unhealthy and healthy approach. A constantly healthy, balanced approach is a *sattvik* attitude.

In order to develop a *sattvik* approach to life, you need to witness your thoughts, observe your actions and continually allow part of your mind to stand back and be the spectator of all your experiences. The act of witnessing yourself is known as **sakshi bhava**. When you are an objective observer then you can see the state/stage of mind you are in. As long as your experiences are subjective, you will be caught in the pain or pleasure of the moment, and nothing else beyond that pain/hurt/anger/jealousy or pleasure can possibly exist.

When negative experiences are stored in your subconscious and unconscious mind you will have negative attitudes. By practising *yoga* techniques your suppressed negative experiences surface and you may be tempted to say, " I don't like *yoga* because it makes me feel angry...it scares me...it makes me feel unsafe..." or, on the other hand, you might say, "*Yoga* is fantastic, I feel full of energy, happy, relaxed". *Yoga* digs out the experiences from within your deeper layers. You need to witness these experiences because they change, everything in life changes, except the *sakshi* witnesser and the Goddess you are seeking. Be the witnesser and you will see the goddessness within yourself also.

In order to reach a state of *yoga* union between mind and spirit/consciousness, you have to develop the awareness of the separation between the two and that they are two different aspects, just as mind and body are two different aspects of you as a whole. The part of you which stands back and observes, the witnesser, is the closest aspect of your mind to spirit/consciousness. We develop this state of awareness in **yoga nidra**™, *pratyahara* sense withdrawal, *dharana* concentration, and so it becomes instilled throughout *dhyana* meditation.

There are many different forms of meditation practice depending on your inclination. Some people are more visual and enjoy imagining scenes. Other people prefer to conjure a particular feeling to achieve mental concentration. Yet others can concentrate easily by remembering particular words, sounds or mantra. The easiest way to gradually focus your mind and develop the art of witnessing is by doing some simple *yoga asana* postures followed by *pranayama* breathing techniques and then *yoga nidra*™ relaxation. When you practise a regular routine of *yoga* techniques you assist the body and mind to evolve out of the *tamasik* and *rajasik* characteristics.

*Hatha yoga* is an easy approach to resolving negative patterns. It is also important to have a network of understanding health care practitioners and friends to support you through negative phases when emotional and psychological cleansing occurs. Through the practices of *Hatha yoga* you not only cleanse your physical body but also the *prana* energy and mental layers as well. While these layers are trying to re-establish their equilibrium you will be undergoing a number of obvious physical and subtle changes. Your experiences of cleansing will vary depending on what has been buried and stored within your subconscious and unconscious layers, within your physical body itself and nervous system, within your *pranik* body and *chakra* energy centres.

## Social Attitudes: *Yama*

*Yoga* is a way of life which assists in your evolution from animal instincts towards divine realization through personal attitudes to yourself, others and your environment. By cultivating **yama** observances you are instilling five important virtues of character which are the expression of a purified mind.

*Ahimsa* is non-violence towards yourself, others, your environment, the earth and the universe. *Ahimsa* also implies non-aggression or non-abusiveness. How many times have you dumped emotional rubbish on someone you love? How many times have you taken advantage of people? Or made a doormat of yourself for others to manipulate? Perhaps you drink a bit too much alcohol or smoke? Don't condemn yourself, rather be more aware of where you gain your self-esteem and what motivates your actions. When you hurt inside, then you will be hurtful to others. By developing a deeper awareness of your thoughts and actions through meditation *ahimsa* will spontaneously unfold. Think of your body and mind as your infant child and take care of your mind and body as you would your child. In this way you will cultivate respect for yourself and others by realizing that the same Self which manifests in you is present in everything. Practise **swadhyaya** which is described below.

*Satya* is truthfulness to yourself and others. This means accepting who you are and how you are and taking respon-

sibility for your thoughts and actions. It doesn't mean telling someone they are horrible just because you think that way when you are depressed and angry. Being truthful would be to say, "I am depressed and angry and everything seems horrible to me." When you are true to yourself you have self-respect and self-esteem. Then you can't be manipulated either. You may find yourself being forced to do something you don't need to do, so you say, "I'm not sure about that." Take time to think about what you want to say and how you are going to say it. If a telemarketer rings you on the phone and you don't want to talk, tell them, "I'm not interested" or "I can't help you". When you are being pressured to make an instant decision then insist on time to think it over. Many sales people tell you that this is a once only offer and you must buy the product or service immediately or you will miss out. This is a marketing ploy and, unless you take time to consider your options, you are going to be untrue to yourself. No one can make you do anything when you are being true to yourself and say what you need to say.

*Asteya* is honesty towards yourself and others. Being honest means not being deceptive or in denial. Be honest to yourself first and then you will want to be honest to others. If you are wrong admit it to yourself first and then learn to say what you did or said was incorrect, "I made a mistake." No need to blame, judge or criticise others because these attitudes are acts of aggression and abuse. If you are angry about a situation say, "I am angry", not, "You make me angry." And again look at yourself. You are angry because that person is not doing what you want them to do. They are not being neat, or they are clumsy, or slow at learning, or .... all the things you don't like. Learn to say, "That's my problem, not yours." In order to be honest you need to look at and accept your fears, insecurities, guilt and shame as well as your strengths and beauty. Realize you are human, you are fallible and you are just as important in the scheme of things as the next person.

*Brahmacharya* is recognizing the same life essence in all beings irrespective of gender. Quite often *brahmacharya* is understood only as abstaining from sexual acts and thoughts. Actually, the word *brahmacharya* means being in the ultimate state with Brahma, the Creator and Universal Spirit. Therefore, true *brahmacharya* is not having sexual feelings for any living being because all you experience is unconditional love and compassion. To practice *brahmacharya* means you are abstaining from sexual activity.

*Aparigraha* is not accumulating what is unnecessary. Have what is necessary for your survival and work in life. Try to let go of all the junk that clutters your cupboards, shelves and drawers. Ultimately you need to clear out the unnecessary emotions and attachments.

## Personal Attitudes: *Niyama*

*Saucha* is cleanliness. Without being neurotic, keep your body clean internally and externally, as well as your house and garden. Uncleanliness breeds germs physically and mentally.

*Santosha* is contentment of mind and emotions. Developing contentment while striving to reach goals may seem contradictory. Goals keep us motivated in life; however, by developing contentment within yourself it checks greed from becoming uncontrollable. Always ask yourself, "Am I being greedy?" And if you are, try to let go of that object. Live within your means, physically and emotionally, and be joyous for what you have got. When you are content, you will be truly happy and able to enjoy your life. *Santosha* also arises by developing dispassion **vairagya** and dispassion can only arise when you are not affected by your feelings of attraction **raga** and repulsion **dwesha**. As long as you prefer one thing above another you cannot experience contentment. By learning to let go of your thoughts and desires you will gravitate towards dispassion and contentment.

*Tapas* is austerity. The more you do without personally, the more you realize you can do without. There is no end to austerity *tapas*, just as there is no end to acquiring. *Tapas* is a good way to fire your body and mind, like firing clay in a kiln. Be moderate while living a simple and balanced lifestyle with abundant love in your heart.

*Swadhyaya* is self-reflection. Take time to reflect on your actions and thoughts. And most importantly develop the ability to witness yourself. The witnesser within you can observe all the different aspects of your mind, your actions and reactions; the personality, intellect, memories, the chatter, emotions, psyche, intuitive knowledge. Also read books about human behavior, co-dependency and addiction and understand your own patterns.

*Ishwara pranidhana* is surrendering to a higher force than your own will. You can change only a few things in your life like your house, your clothes, your car, even your wife or husband! However, there are some things in life that cannot be changed and, the sooner you let go of your resistance, the easier life is. You have grown up knowing that the sun rises in the morning and sets in the evening. You do not try to change sunrise or sunset because it would be futile and a waste of time and energy. Therefore, you work around sunrise and sunset. So why do you struggle with everything else and everyone else? Life may have dealt you heavy blows. Consider these as lessons for your personal growth. You can use these experiences to make yourself a stronger and better person. When you develop *santosha, swadhyaya* and live simply, then *Ishwara Pranidhana* will unfold spontaneously.

**Every person comes into this world with 4 basic desires that have to be fulfilled; *kama, artha, dharma* and *moksha*.**

*Kama* is defined as sensual pleasure. It is the desire to touch or be touched either non sexually or sexually.

*Artha* is the need to acquire material possessions and wealth.

*Dharma* is your desire to follow a profession and lifestyle that fits in with your character.

*Moksha* is freedom and self-realization. The desire for freedom and self-knowledge often remains dormant for quite some time before it gradually surfaces. When you feel limited and restricted by your circumstances and strive for a way to free yourself, you are experiencing the need for moksha. It also surfaces when you start to question who you really are and what is your relation to the world you live in. Most likely you started to experience the need for *moksha* at puberty and perhaps later during your forties.

There are some people who also need fame. This desire really is an aggregate of all the four basic needs. If one of your needs is not being met then you will crave it. The majority of people have a strong craving for sensual pleasure and objects of enjoyment while the last two desires of *dharma* and *moksha* are less predominant. Applying one or more of the *yama* and *niyama* will help you to keep these four basic needs in balance.

# CHAPTER THREE

# Cleansing Practices

*Clarity of mind,*
*purity of emotion,*
*cleanliness of body and habits,*
*lightness of heart and generosity*
*will set your spirit free.*

(Muktibodha)

Depending on where and when you were born your society has varying ideas about marriage, food, dress, family, work, etc. and so you are born into a certain mind set. The ramifications of living in a particular society are both psychological and physiological, both positive and negative. Specific cleansing practices are known to relieve physical and mental stress. When you service your car you can drive it safely; when you clean out your cupboards you can see what is inside; when you resolve troublesome problems you can sleep well. And when you purge your body of toxins you can function healthily on all levels.

There are popular methods of internal cleansing these days using herbs, teas, juices, enemas and fasting. Whatever

your method of cleansing, be informed about the process, the consequences and what will suit your individual needs.

## Fasting

The most balanced approach to fasting is to eat a fruitarian diet for the day and include either milk or yogurt and water. That's it, just fruit, milk or yogurt and water, no soya products or grains, no tea of any sort, coffee, salt, sugar, spices, condiments, tobacco, etc., etc. Fasting should be done with a specific moon date and phase not just because you ate too much last night or you want to lose weight.

A lunar month consists of two phases, one when the moon is waxing and becoming fuller and the other when the moon is waning and becoming smaller. Each phase is divided into 15 parts which are not equivalent to the 24-hour day/night date. The first day after full moon is the first day of the dark fortnight or waning moon phase. The first day after no moon is day one of the bright fortnight or waxing moon phase. For optimum results from fasting it is best to choose either the fourth, seventh, ninth, 11th, full moon or no moon dates during the waxing or waning moon phase.

Alternatively you can fast on a specific day of the week corresponding to a particular planet in your natal astrological chart that brings in disturbing energy. Sunday is ruled by the sun, monday by the moon, tuesday by mars, wednesday by mercury, thursday by jupiter, friday by venus and saturday by saturn. If you don't have a natal chart but have observed that your worst times often occur on a particular day, then make that your fasting day.

## Tantric Nyasa

In the system of *tantra* cleansing of the physical and subtle bodies is accomplished through touching specific body parts and applying ash made from cow manure while repeating an appropriate *mantra* sound. This is known as **nyasa**. It literally means 'placing' or 'depositing'. By practising *nyasa* you replace negative energy patterns with positive ones. The purpose of *nyasa* is to prepare you for meditation so that the energy produced from the practice can flow freely through your body and mind.

There are different varieties of *nyasa*.

Here is one example:

Touch the forehead with ring and middle fingers while repeating:
*Aum Am Namaha*

Touch the upper and lower lips with the index, middle and ring fingers while repeating:
*Aum Em Namaha, Aum Aiym Namaha*

Touch the eyes right and left with the thumb and ring fingers while repeating:
*Aum Im Namaha, Aum Im Namaha*

Touch the ears right and left with the thumb while repeating:
*Aum Um Namaha, Aum Um Namaha*

Touch the nostrils right and left with the thumb and little fingers while repeating:
*Aum Rim Namaha, Aum Rim Namaha*

Touch the cheeks right and left with the index, middle and ring fingers while repeating:
*Aum Lrim Namaha, Aum Lrim Namaha*

Touch the crown of head with the middle fingers while repeating:
*Aum Am Namaha*

Point inside the mouth with the ring and middle fingers while repeating:
*Aum Ah Namaha*

Touch from the heart to the right leg with the little, ring and middle fingers while repeating:
*Aum Sam Namaha*

Touch from the heart to the left leg with the little, ring and middle fingers while repeating:
*Aum Ham Namaha*

Touch the back with the little, ring and middle fingers while repeating:
*Aum Bam Namaha*

Touch the navel with the little, ring and middle fingers and thumb while repeating:
*Aum Ram Namaha*

Touch the right shoulder with the palm while repeating:
*Aum Ram Namaha*

Touch the left shoulder with the palm while repeating:
*Aum Ram Namaha*

Touch the shoulder centre and neck base with the palm while repeating:
*Aum Lam Namaha*

## Hatha Yoga Shat Karma
### six internal cleansing practices
These practices should be done only under expert guidance.

*Neti* is the practice of cleaning the nasal passages either with saline water **jala neti** or a thread/catheter **sutra neti.** For *jala neti* a special *neti* pot is used to pour the water through your nostrils. *Neti* must be learnt under the guidance of an experienced teacher.

*Dhauti* is a general name given to various internal cleansing practices such as cleaning the mouth, ears and entire alimentary canal. To clean the alimentary canal there are 2 practices, one is abbreviated the other is not.

DHAUTI MUST BE LEARNT UNDER THE GUIDANCE OF AN EXPERIENCED TEACHER.

For the abbreviated version **laghu shankha prakshalana** you drink a total of six glasses of saline water. In-between each two glasses of water five different *asana* postures are practised to flush the water through your system.
When practising the full version **purna shankhaprakshalan** you drink 16 glasses of warm saline water, interspersed by the same *asana* postures as the abbreviated version. After drinking 16 glasses of saline water there is dietary restric-

tion to restore the lining of the digestive system.

*Nauli* is the control, isolation and churning of the abdominal muscles.

*Basti* is a technique to wash the large intestine by sucking up water through the anal passage, something like an enema, however you have to be adept in the practice of *nauli*.

*Kapalbhati* is rapid breathing through the nose to stimulate the frontal brain lobes. Exhalation is emphasized in *kapalbhati*, inhalation is the result of the forced exhalation.

*Trataka* is gazing steadily at an object such as a single point or candle flame in order to still the rapid eye movements.

## *Sphatika Shuddhi* **cleansing with crystals**

Cleansing your internal energy system can be achieved using quartz crystals. Quartz crystal possesses piezoelectric[*] properties and, by rubbing a crystal on your body or surrounding yourself with crystals, you can clear energy blockages as well as increase your energy supply. Refer to Chapter 8 for the description of the practice.

---

[*]The Greek word *piezein* means to press or squeeze. Piezoelectricity is so called because it is electricity produced from a specific class of crystalline material under compression. The crystalline structure of quartz produces a voltage proportional to the applied pressure. Due to this property of piezoelectricity, quartz crystal has many uses in modern technology, such as in radios, televisions, watches, lasers, photovoltaic cells and computers.

# CHAPTER FOUR

# Body stabilization: *Asana*

*Asana is spoken of as the first part of Hatha yoga before everything else.*
*Having performed asana one attains steadiness of body and mind diseaselessness and flexibility of limbs.*

(*Hatha Yoga Pradipika:* Chapter 1 verse 17)

Most people today feel pushed by a modern lifestyle. As a result of the hectic pace of life you may experience poor health and stress, and find that prescribed medicine does not completely alleviate your symptoms. At this point you will start to search for a way to help yourself. *Yoga* techniques can enable you to resolve most of your physical, emotional, mental and spiritual stress. While you may not be able to make the stressful situations go away, you can certainly improve your ability to manage yourself and cope.

*Hatha yoga* assists in regaining inner equilibrium of the body which reflects in the mind and emotions. It is a systematic process of balancing the production of hormonal secretions and nervous impulses through the body and brain. A carefully designed *yoga* program is essential for each person. Finding a local *yoga* class these days is usually easy. However, finding a *yoga* teacher that can instruct according to your individual needs may be more challenging.

There are different styles of *yoga* being taught, ranging from gentle to gymnastic. The physical practices come under the broad term *Hatha yoga;* however, the different styles being taught now are often named according to the prominent teacher. Whatever style or lineage of *yoga* you practise the *yoga asana* postures should essentially give you both physical core strength as well as flexibility. If you do not gain core strength you can become too flexible, or if you gain too much strength then you will lose flexibility. Be aware of your individual needs and ask questions about the style of *yoga* to determine if it is what you are looking for.

The word *asana* (pronounced aa-sun-a) indicates a steady and comfortable position of your body that can promote the state of meditation. It is preferable to perform the *yoga asana* slowly and maintain the final position for 30 seconds to a minute. When you practise quickly you cannot feel each part of your body involved in the *asana*. It is also advisable to practise according to your health status. Some *asana* postures may be contradictory to your present state of health. For example, if you have high blood pressure you should not lower your head down below your heart. Or during pregnancy you should not bend backwards as it accentuates the spinal

curvature. Also avoid backward bending if you have a hernia or stomach ulcer. Do not attempt inverted poses if you have a brain tumor. In fact, inverted postures should be learnt only under the expert guidance of a teacher.

There are various precautions you need to be aware of when you have a health concern. While the *asana* practices described here are safe and health promoting you should always consult your health care practitioner before commencing.

## When, where and how

*Asana* is practised on an empty stomach, never after eating, except for the sitting posture of *vajrasana* which enhances the digestive power. The traditional way of eating in Japan employs *vajrasana*, sitting on the shins. If you have varicose veins, however, this pose is not suitable. It is preferable to practise *yoga* in the morning, however, if it is not possible, limit the amount of dynamic *asana* postures you do at night otherwise you won't be able to sleep. *Yoga* is invigorating. When you practise in the evening do *asana* postures that are calming and save the dynamic practices for the morning. Wear loose comfortable clothing that does not restrict your movement and remove excess jewelry. *Yoga* is about simplicity; keep your lifestyle simple; diet simple; requirements simple and clothing simple.

There are various 'yoga props' that can be bought. Use whatever is essential to your practice. It is unnecessary to buy props and gear until you commence and find out exactly what you do need. Use clothes and blankets made of natural fibres if possible, to allow the earth's electromagnetic fields to flow through you. This also means practising on a blanket of natural fibre. If you are practising on a hard floor you will need a mat that doesn't slip. A folded blanket can be useful for supporting you in certain postures and you will need it for sitting on during *pranayama* breathing and meditation. Keeping in mind that *asana* means a steady and comfortable position, if you are not comfortable then you are not practising *yoga asana* postures. Understand the difference between stretching and straining. Be aware of the part of your body that is being stretched. Mentally communicate with your body and encourage it to relax, let go into the stretch, relax, relax, relax. Certain parts of the body need to be tensed to hold you in position, let go of all the other parts that don't need to be tensed. *Asana* postures lead to slow careful movements, controlled by deep regular breathing. Use your breath to facilitate the movement, inhalation for stretching, exhalation for relaxing and letting go, breath retention or gentle breathing for holding the position.

Prior to any major *asana*, commence with preparatory *asana* postures that stretch all your muscles. Preliminary *asana* practices are the most useful because they also work on many muscle groups, improve and regulate your circulation, nervous system, digestive system

and hormonal secretions from the glands. There is a lot of information these days describing various *yoga asana* postures. According to the ancient *Hatha Yoga Pradipika* text there are as many *asana* postures as there are forms of life. The following series is specifically designed for men and women to enhance the endocrine system, digestive system and organs, spine and skeletal system, joints, muscles, nervous system, reproductive organs and brain. If any of the *asana* postures are unsuitable for you, do not practise them. However, you can receive benefit by visualizing or imagining yourself performing those particular *asana* postures. Choose the *asana* postures according to the areas of your body that need attention.

**Practise in the given sequence in the following pages, always commencing with *shavasana* for a minute.**

## 1. *Shavasana* corpse relaxation pose:

Relax supine, with your feet apart, arms away from your body, palms turned upward, legs, spine and head are in alignment, lower jaw relaxed, upper and lower teeth slightly separated and your tongue relaxed behind the lower teeth. Let go of all resistance. In a few moments feel as if your body is melting into the floor.

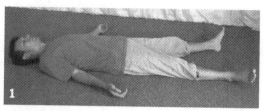

## 2. Leg lock pose from *Supta pawan muktasana* series:

Continue lying supine, keep your legs together and whole body in alignment. Draw your right knee towards your chest while leaving the left leg relaxed on the floor. Clasp your fingers around or under your knee.

While gradually exhaling, raise your head towards your knee and gently squeeze your thigh towards your abdomen. Hold still for a moment allowing the hip to relax. Be aware of any pressure on the right side of your abdomen. Inhale slowly while releasing. Practise five to 10 times.

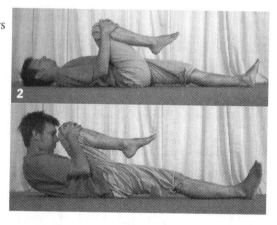

Next, keep your knee bent and place your right hand on top of your knee. Rotate the whole leg clockwise five to 10 times and then anticlockwise.

Repeat the whole process with the left leg.

Practise leg lock pose with both legs together five to eight times.

While your knees are at your chest, hold your knees with your hands, right hand on the right knee, left hand on the left knee. Circle your legs in the same direction, being aware of your lower back massaging against the floor. Practise five to eight rotations in one direction and then reverse it. Be aware of your hips, abdomen and the lower back. This movement is very soothing for the lower back and abdomen.

### 3. *Supta mandirashira ayam asana* **hamstring stretch pose:**

Keep your knees bent and place your feet on the floor in front of your buttocks. Lift your right leg straight up into the air and clasp your hands behind the back of your leg wherever comfortable. Keep the right knee as straight as possible while drawing the leg closer to you. If you find it difficult to straighten the knee, place one hand behind your knee and the other on the kneecap giving you more support. You can place one

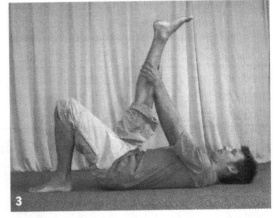

hand behind your knee and the other on the kneecap to help straighten your knee. As you gain flexibility, relax your left leg on the floor while stretching your right leg in the air. Keep your leg raised and continue onto the next movement.

### 4. *Supta ghuti avritti* **lying ankle rotation:**

Holding your leg in the air without stretching the hamstring, slowly rotate your foot in one direction and then the other.

Then practise **3.** *supta mandirashirayam asana* and **4.** *supta ghuti avritti* with the left leg.

## 5. *Nitambayamasana* **gluteus maximus stretch:**

Place a folded blanket under your head and shoulders for this *asana*. Keep your left foot on the floor close to your buttock and rest your right ankle above your left knee. Bring your left leg towards you and clasp your hands behind the back of your left thigh, or around the outside of your left shin. As you carefully draw your left leg inwards you will feel your right gluteus maximus stretching. If it is very uncomfortable try straightening the left leg in the air while drawing the leg closer to you. Hold for 30 seconds or so while focusing on relaxing any tightness you may feel in your leg. Slowly release and practise in the same way with the left leg.

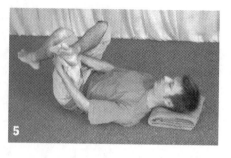

## 6. *Saral chakrasana* **wheel pose preparation:**

Place your feet on the floor close to your buttocks keeping them hip width apart. Stretch your arms above your head. If you cannot rest your arms comfortably on the floor, bend your elbows and hold your forearms, or simply keep them by the sides of your body. Inhale gradually while lifting your pelvis. Remain in this *asana* posture while retaining your breath, or alternatively breathe gently and hold the pose for 30 seconds or so. Be aware of all the areas of your body that are affected, such as your thighs, pelvis, abdomen, lower back, torso slightly inverted, perhaps a slight pressure in the throat, the stretch in the area of your cervical spine. Practise for 30 to 60 seconds. When you release, relax down gradually while exhaling. Keep your arms stretched above your head, legs straight on the floor. Inhale slowly stretching your whole body, exhale and relax your arms by your sides again. Practise for 30 to 60 seconds.

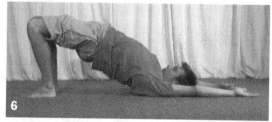

Lie in *shavasana* **corpse relaxation pose** for 30 seconds.

### 7. *Poorwa halasana* **plough pose preparation:**

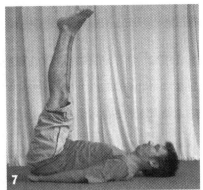

Bring your knees towards your chest. Place your hands underneath your rump keeping the palms against the floor. Now make fists with your hands to give a little height under your lower back. Lift your legs up into the air and angle them towards you. Remain in this asana as long as comfortable. Be aware of the whole position your body. When you release the pose, flatten your hands to the floor, bend your knees and place your feet on the floor. Place your hands by your sides again and slide your legs down to the floor.

Lie in *shavasana* **corpse relaxation pose** for 30 seconds.

### 8. *Pada kalavartasana* **leg cycling** based on *supta pawan muktasana:*

Bring your knees to your chest and tuck your hands under your rump area, palms turned downward. Cycle your legs around as if you are riding a bicycle in slow motion and feel all the muscles involved. To challenge yourself, do it even more slowly and stretch your legs out towards the floor.

Alternatively, if it is uncomfortable cycling with both legs simultaneously, practise cycling one leg at a time. While cycling your right leg, place your left foot on the floor close to your buttock. Cycle clockwise and anti clockwise and then change legs.

Depending on your level of fitness, you may need to relax before reversing the cycling movements.

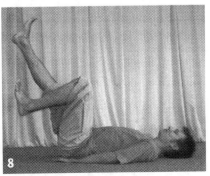

Practise five to 20 rotations in each direction and then change legs.

This is an excellent practice to gain joint flexibility in your knees and hips and to strengthen the thighs, abdomen, lower back and psoas* muscles. It also influences the digestive system.

### 9. *Supta pada ayamasana* **lying leg stretch:**

Either lift your legs vertically and then angle them towards you or bend your knees to your chest. Take hold of your big toes if possible, or hold your legs wherever comfortable. Keep your knees as straight as possible. Slowly separate your legs, relaxing your inner thighs and hamstrings. Hold the final position for 30 seconds or so. Slowly release the *asana* the same way as you came into it. During pregnancy you can practise with your legs against the wall, without holding your toes. Any posture with your legs raised benefits the valves in your leg veins. In this position the blood flows through the valves more easily, assisted by gravity as it returns to the heart.

### 10. *Supta samavrit vanshasana* **spinal twist**

**Stage one:**
Stretch your arms out shoulder height on the floor with your palms turned downward. Alternatively, you can interlace your fingers behind the back of your neck. Bend your knees and place your feet on the floor. Keep your knees and feet together and slowly inhale. This is the base position for *supta samavrit vansha-asana.* While exhaling gradually, lower your legs as far as possible towards the floor on the right. Breathe normally while maintaining the spinal twist and be aware of your back and spine. Then inhale gradually while bringing your legs back to the centre. Practise on the other side. Repeat five to 10 times.

---

*psoas muscles are large muscles that emanate from the sides of the lumbar spine and fit into the upper end of the thigh bones. The psoas muscles assist the spine to be upright. If they are constantly engaged, the adrenal glands can be drained.

**Stage two:**

Remain in the base position with your arms spread on the floor, knees bent and feet on the floor.

Gradually inhale while lifting your legs towards your chest and slowly exhale lowering your legs across towards the floor on your right. Place your knees as close as possible towards your right elbow. Remain in the spinal twist breathing normally. Relax into your body position. Then, you can turn your head to the left if it feels comfortable to do so. Be aware of your whole

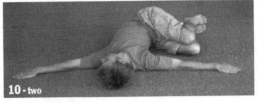

back and spine. Inhale gradually while bringing your legs and head back to the centre. Now practise on the other side. Repeat five to 10 times each side.

**Stage three:**

Practise the second stage keeping your head centred and when you have lowered your legs to the right side start to straighten them until you have reached a comfortable position. Remain in this spinal twist breathing normally and feel the turning of your back and spine. To release your position again bend your knees and inhale gradually raising your legs back to the centre. Perform this *asana* one to three times either side.

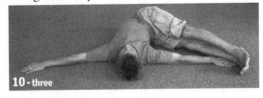

Lie in *shavasana* **corpse relaxation pose** for 30 seconds.

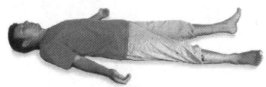

## 11. *Avalambi pada ayamasana* **reclining leg stretch:**

Lie on your left side and bend your left elbow supporting your head in your hand. Balance yourself by placing your right hand on the floor in front of your navel. If you feel uncomfortable lying on your side, place a folded blanket beneath you. Bring both knees towards your right hand.

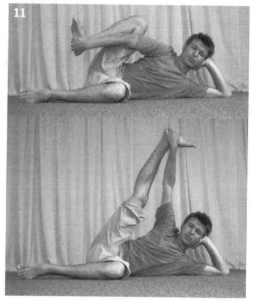

Slowly raise your right knee upwards and hold your instep. Gradually straighten your leg into the air. You may want to bend and stretch your leg a few times to make it easier. Then, as you gain flexibility, grip the ball of your foot and draw your leg towards your head. Maintain the final position for 30 seconds or so. Before practising on the other side, continue with the next *asana*.

## 12. *Chirika asana* **cricket pose:**

Lie on your left side with your left elbow on the floor, left hand supporting your head and your legs straight. Balance yourself by placing your right hand on the floor in front of your navel. Feel comfortable in this base position. If you feel uncomfortable lying on your side, place a folded blanket beneath you. Inhale slowly while bringing your right knee up towards your right arm keeping your leg parallel to the floor. Exhale slowly straightening your leg back behind you a few centimeters, continuing to keep your leg parallel to the floor.

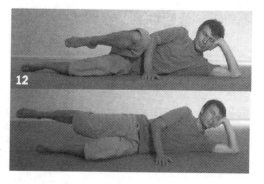

Repeat these movements five to 20 times being aware of the muscles in your thigh, abdomen and lower back.

*12. continues on next page*

After continual practice you will notice these areas become stronger.

On completion lie down on the same side with your left arm stretched on the floor above you. Relax your head on the upper arm and let go for a few moments. This is the base position for the next _asana_.

### 13. _Vishram utthita padasana_ **lying leg lift:**

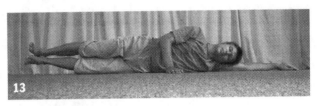

Lying on your left side with your left arm on the floor above your head and right hand on the floor in front of your navel, inhale gradually while lifting both legs simultaneously. Maintain the final position, either retaining your breath or breathe lightly so you can hold longer. As you hold, feel your thighs, abdomen and lower back. Release slowly while exhaling. Practise for 30 seconds or so and then roll onto your back.

_Lie in shavasana_ for a few moments then practise **11, 12,** and **13** on the other side.

### 14. _Advasana_ **one angle pose:**

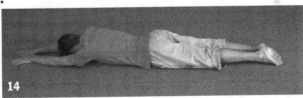

Lie on your abdomen with your arms on the floor above your head. Place your forehead on the floor while tucking your chin in towards your throat. If you cannot breathe easily in this position, rest your forehead on a folded blanket. Your legs and ankles should be kept together. Mentally check the alignment of your legs, spine, head and arms. Let go of all resistance in your body to assist the vertebrae to align themselves.

Relax in this pose for 30 seconds or so.

### 15. _Arari ayamasana_ **diagonal stretch:**

From _advasana,_ inhale gradually while raising your right arm, head and left leg. Pull the right arm forward and the left leg backward while holding for a moment and retaining your breath. Feel the diagonal stretch through your back. Exhale slowly while releasing the posture. Practise on the other side. Perform this _asana_ three to five times.

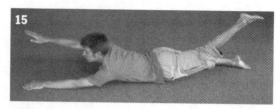

### 16. _Laghu naukasana_ **canoe pose:**

Lying in _advasana,_ inhale slowly while simultaneously raising your arms, head and legs. It is important to keep your feet together and knees straight. You do not need to lift your legs and arms high into the air. Hold the final posture while retaining your breath, or you can challenge yourself by holding longer and breathing gently. Feel into your back, shoulders and neck whilst holding the _asana_ posture. Release on exhalation. Perform this _asana_ three to five times.

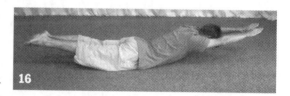

### 17. _Jyestikasana_ **auspicious pose:**

Place your forehead on the floor, and interlace your fingers behind your neck. Keep your legs together in alignment with your spine and head. Relax here for half a minute or so being aware of your back, shoulder blade and neck areas. Let go of all resistance in your body to assist the vertebrae to align themselves.

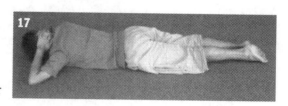

## 18. *Tarana makarasana* **swimming crocodile:**

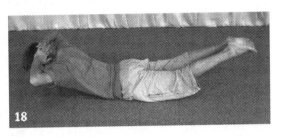

From the base position of *jyesti-kasana* rest your hands behind the back of your head. Gradually inhale while lifting your arms, head, and legs simultaneously. If this is not possible then slightly raise your arms only. Maintain the final position while retaining your breath or breathe gently to hold longer. Be aware of the areas in your back and shoulders that are affected. Also feel the buttocks tensing. Slowly exhale as you release. Practise for half a minute or so and repeat two to three times.

This form of backward bending assists in strengthening the pelvic floor muscles. *Tarana makarasana* posture may be practised during the first few weeks of pregnancy.

## 19. *Nidran makarasana* **sleeping crocodile:**

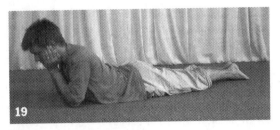

Relax on your abdomen placing your elbows on the floor and chin in the palms. Keep your elbows close together and towards your chest. Your neck should not extend backwards. As you relax in *nidran makarasana* take your awareness to the gentle bend of your lower back. Relax in the posture for half a minute or so. If you have a slipped disc or sciatica it may be beneficial to practise frequently, remaining in the position for a few minutes. It can be practiced during the first few weeks of pregnancy.

### 20. *Uddi shalabhasana* **flying locust:**

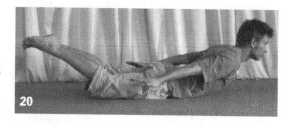

Keep your forehead on the floor and place your hands about 30 centimeters (12") away from your sides with the palms turned downward.

Your legs remain together throughout the practice. Gradually inhale while lifting your head, arms and legs. As you hold the pose, pull your arms towards the wall behind you and either retain your breath or breathe gently to hold longer. Focus your awareness in the spine, back muscles, shoulders and neck. Release slowly while exhaling. Practise for half a minute or so. If you have a back problem, perform this *asana* daily. It may be performed during the first few weeks of pregnancy.

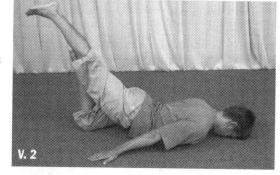

#### Variation two:
From your base position, bend your left knee and lift your right leg while inhaling. Rest your right knee on the sole of your left foot. Be aware of your lower back and make sure that you are not rotating the right hip outward. Breathe normally and hold for half a minute or so being aware of the bend in your back. Practise on the other side. Perform this asana once or twice. Strong backward bending should be avoided after the first few weeks of pregnancy.

### 21. *Shalabhasana* **locust pose:**

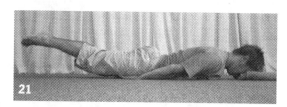

Lying on your abdomen with your forehead on the floor, tuck your hands underneath your thighs with the palms against your body. If your arms are not comfortable, place them close by your sides with your palms against the floor. Keep your legs together and mentally check your alignment. Gradually inhale while raising your legs. Keep your knees straight and feet together. If you cannot lift both legs simultaneously, then raise one leg at a time. Hold the final position while retaining your breath. Alternatively, breathe gently so you can maintain the posture for a longer period. As you hold the final position be aware of your lower back. Release slowly while exhaling. Perform this *asana* three to five times.

If you practise this *asana* daily your lower back and pelvic floor muscles will become stronger.

### 22. *Sarpasana* snake pose:

Lying in the same base position with your forehead on the floor, interlace your fingers behind your lower back or hold one wrist with the opposite hand.

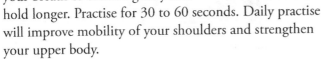

Your legs should remain together on the floor throughout the *asana*. Inhale gradually while raising your head and pulling your arms towards the wall behind you. You may either hold the posture while retaining your breath or breathe gently and hold longer. Practise for 30 to 60 seconds. Daily practise will improve mobility of your shoulders and strengthen your upper body.

### 23. *Saral bhujangasana* easy cobra pose:

DO NOT ATTEMPT THIS ASANA IF YOU HAVE A HERNIA OR STOMACH ULCER.

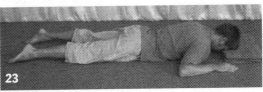

Place your forehead on the floor with your hands beneath your shoulders, palms against the floor. Next, slide your hands forward until they are either side of your face. Separate your legs in alignment with your hips. Place the top of your feet on the floor. This is the

*23 continues next page*

base position for *saral bhujangasana*. Gradually inhale while guiding your chin forward and raising your head and chest. Let your hands and arms support your upper body as you lift. Only straighten your arms if possible and keep your neck upright. Hold the posture feeling the bend in your lower back. Check that your shoulders do not lift up around your ears, that your pubic bone is touching the floor and buttocks are relaxed. While holding this *asana* you can retain the breath or hold longer by breathing gently. Practise this *asana* three to five times.

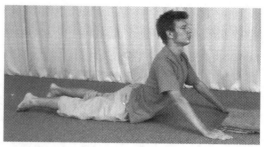

Backward bending may increase bleeding during menstruation so you may decide not to practise it during that time.

### 24. *Tulit dhanurasana* balanced bow pose:

DO NOT ATTEMPT THIS ASANA IF YOU HAVE A HERNIA OR STOMACH ULCER.

Place your forehead on the floor with your left arm stretched above your head and right arm by your side. Bend your left knee and clasp the top of your left foot with your right hand. Alternatively, bend the right knee and hold the right foot with the right hand. Gradually inhale while simultaneously lifting your head and thigh. Create resistance between your hand and foot. The arm above your head should remain on the floor. Be aware of your right shoulder, chest, back and any other area you feel this *asana* affecting. Hold the final pose either retaining your breath or breathing gently. Practise one to three times. Release, relax and then practise on the other side.

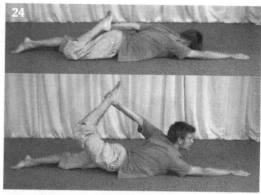

As backward bending can increase blood flow during menstruation, you may prefer not to practise this *asana* at that time.

### 25. *Visphur dhanurasana* **bending the bow pose:**

DO NOT ATTEMPT THIS ASANA IF YOU HAVE A
HERNIA OR STOMACH ULCER.

Lie on your abdomen with your
arms by your sides, forehead on the
floor and legs separated. Bend your
knees and grip the top of your feet.
Gradually inhale while simultaneously lifting your head, chest and
thighs. Create resistance between
your hands and feet. Hold as long
as comfortable, either retaining your
breath or breathing gently. Be aware
of the areas affected as you hold the
pose. Alternatively, you can main-

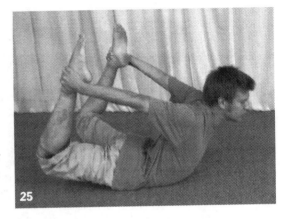

tain awareness from your navel through to your spine.
Release the posture slowly during exhalation. Practise
one to three times.

### 26. *Matsya kridasana* **flapping fish pose:**

Lie on your right side with your arms in front, elbows
bent and hands placed one on top of the other. Rest

your cheek on the
back of your hands.
Bend your left knee
and place your foot
behind the back of
your right leg. Use

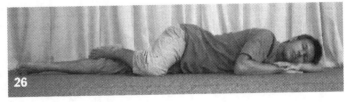

cushions for support under the left thigh and knee,
head and chest areas if you need. During the later stages
of pregnancy always use cushions or folded blankets to
support your body in this posture. You will find it is a
very comfortable pose for your lower back.

Also, when you lie on your right side, your left nostril
will be uppermost, and after some time you will breathe
predominantly through your left nostril. This is conducive for relaxing and falling asleep. Therefore, it is a
suitable position if you suffer from insomnia.

## 27. *Marjari asana* **cat pose:**

Kneel with your hands placed directly beneath your shoulders. Place your palms on the floor. If your wrists are uncomfortable, then make fists and place the knuckles against the floor. Keep your knees in alignment with your hips, feet in alignment with your knees. You may need to kneel on a folded blanket if you have a knee problem.

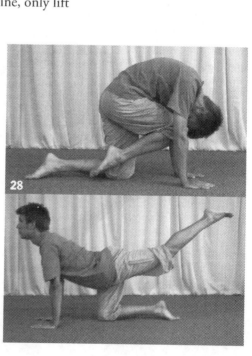

Gradually inhale while moving your head backwards and depressing your back. Slowly exhale while bringing your chin towards your throat, lifting your spine like a cat arching its back and pushing your pelvis forward. Feel your torso as you lift and lower your spine. Practise for half a minute or so.

During pregnancy do not depress your spine, only lift your back as far as possible.

*Marjari asana* massages the inner organs and works on the spine. It is particularly useful for women as it influences the female reproductive system.

## 28. *Vyagrasana* **tiger pose:**

Remain in the same base position of *marjari asana* and place your legs together. Before moving, inhale slowly. Then gradually exhale while lowering your head and lifting your right knee forwards.

Inhale gradually, lifting your head and straightening your right leg backward, and upward if possible. Be aware of the forward and backward bending movements affecting your hip, abdomen, and back.

Practise five to 10 times with each leg.

**Variation two:**

From your base position, inhale gradually and stretch your right leg backwards and upwards while raising your left arm shoulder height. Hold. Exhale slowly as you release. Now practise on the other side. Be aware of all movements and areas of your body that are affected. Practise three to 10 times each side.

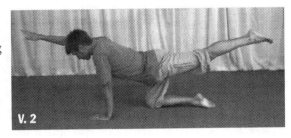

### 29. *Parvatasana* **mountain pose:**

DO NOT PERFORM THIS ASANA IF YOU HAVE HIGH BLOOD PRESSURE.

Remain in the same base position of *vyagrasana* and turn your toes under so the balls of your feet are against the floor. Inhale slowly lifting your knees and straightening your legs, push your heels down towards the floor. Let your head hang between your arms. Try to straighten your back. Remain in this position breathing gently. Be aware of the blood flowing into your head, the stretch through your hamstrings and Achilles tendons and your lower back and abdomen relaxing. Hold for 30 seconds or so. Inhale slowly and lift your head. Then gradually exhale while bending your knees to the floor.

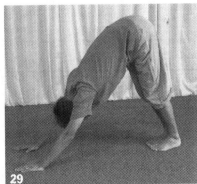

Sit in *vajrasana* for a few moments with your eyes closed and focus on the breath in your nostrils. Perform this asana two or three times.

### 30. *Bhumi bhalamasana* **forehead to ground pose:**

DO NOT PERFORM THIS <u>A</u>SANA IF YOU HAVE
HIGH BLOOD PRESSURE.

Remain in the same base position of *vya-grasana* and turn your fingers inwards. With
your head up, inhale slowly. While exhaling
lower your forehead to the floor and keep
your bottom in the air. Breathe gently and
remain in the final pose for a few moments.
Be aware of your lower back and abdomen
relaxing; the inversion of your torso; the
sensation around your shoulder blades and
blood flowing into your head. Inhale slowly
while lifting up into the base position. Practise this *<u>a</u>sana* two or three times.

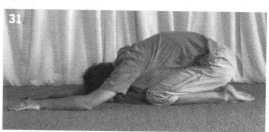

### 31. *Shashankasana* **moon pose:**

IF YOU HAVE HIGH BLOOD PRESSURE
DO NOT LOWER YOUR HEAD BELOW
YOUR HEART.

Sit in *vajrasana* (see ahead, pg. 54, #36) and inhale
slowly lifting your arms above your head. Exhale slowly
and bend forward from your hips. Place your hands on
the floor first and slide down until
your forehead relaxes on the floor.

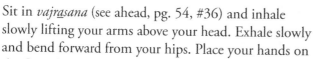

Alternatively, placing your forehead
on the floor, you may like to bring
your arms beside your body with
your palms turned upward. This
opens up the shoulder blade area.

If you cannot lower your head down, rest your elbows
on the floor and chin in your hands. You may need to
separate your knees if there is too much pressure in the
abdomen.

Relax in the *<u>a</u>sana* for 30 seconds or so.

When releasing your position, raise your head and then sit up slowly inhaling while stretching your arms above your head. As you exhale lower your hands towards your knees.

*Shashankasana* has a relaxing effect on the body and mind and is useful if you suffer from insomnia; it may assist in relieving an asthmatic attack and it affects the female reproductive system.

## 32. *Pawan muktasana* **for your feet and knees:**

Sit with your legs stretched in front. Place your hands either side of you on the floor and lift your bottom up then lower yourself down. Now place your hands on your legs. Alternatively, you can sit with your lower back against the wall. This is your base position.

Now gently squeeze your toes away from you and then pull them back, separating them. Be aware of the spaces between your toes as you draw them back. Practise for half a minute or so.

Next point your feet away from you and flex them back. Be aware of all the movements in the feet and ankles.

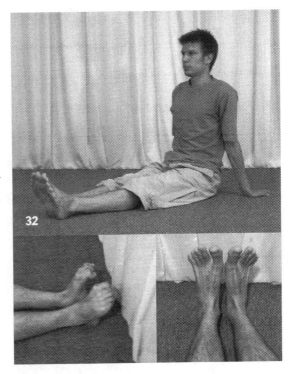

These movements are beneficial to your toe joints, ankles, feet muscles, circulation and co-ordination.

*32 continues next page*

Bend your right knee and hold your forearms under your leg or interlace your fingers. Keep your foot off the floor while slowly rotating your lower leg five to eight times in one direction and then the other. Be aware of your knee and thigh muscles. Practise with the other leg in the same way.

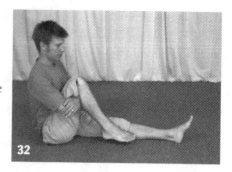

### 33. *Tiryaka sukhasana* sideways bending sitting pose:

Sit cross-legged and interlace your fingers in your lap. Inhale slowly lifting your hands above your head, palms turned upward and exhale slowly lowering your hands behind your head. Pull your shoulder blades closer together inhaling.

Exhale slowly bending to your right, bringing your elbow towards your knee or calf muscle. To challenge yourself take your right elbows across to the left knee. Inhale slowly while coming up to a sitting position and then exhale bending to the other side. Be aware of your body while bending, turning and lifting. Practise five to eight times on both sides.

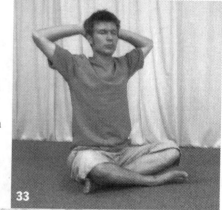

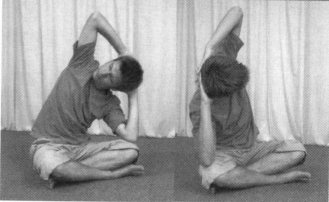

## 34. *Ardha vatayamasana* **half groin stretch:**

From a cross-legged position stretch your left leg out sideways. Place both hands on the floor in front of you.

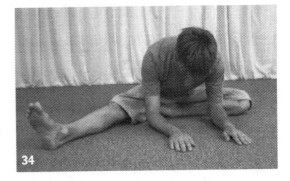

Inhale slowly and looking straight ahead, exhale gradually sliding your hands forward and bringing your forearms to the floor. Look at the floor and bounce gently, while breathing normally.

Then inhale slowly and raise your head sitting upright. Practise on the other side.

## 35. *Upavishta parivritasana* **seated turning pose:**

Remain in your base position with your left leg stretched sideways. Place your hands on your knees and lift up from your lower back while inhaling.

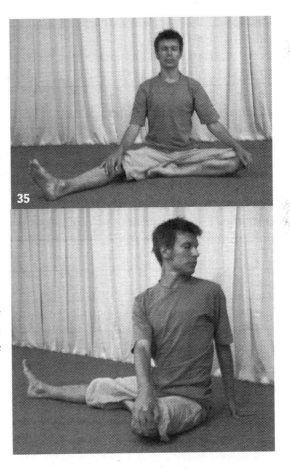

Exhale slowly and turn to the right, placing your right behind you and left hand on the right knee. Breathe normally and allow your legs to relax. Be aware of the turning of your spine. Take your awareness to your eyebrow centre, **bhru madhya**. This is the external focal point corre-lating to the top of your spine. Hold half a minute or so and then practise on the other side.

### 36. *Vajrāsana* **lightning pose:**

DO NOT PERFORM THIS ASANA IF YOU HAVE
VARICOSE VEINS OR A KNEE PROBLEM.

Kneel on your shins, placing your right big toe over your
left big toe. Your heels turn sideways and you sit on the
soles of your feet. You may need to place a folded blanket
or cushion between your feet and buttocks to reduce any
pressure. Rest your palms on your thighs towards your
knees. Remain in *vajrāsana* for 30 seconds or so. Close
your eyes and focus your mind on the flow of breath in
your nostrils. You may feel the breath is flowing more
obviously through one nostril than the other. Sometimes
the breath seems to flow evenly through both nostrils.

*Vajrāsana* is recommended during pregnancy and to ease
lower back pain. It may also assist relieving heartburn
and promote digestion after eating.

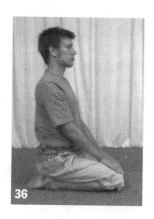

### 37. *Pawan muktāsana* **for the hands and arms:**

Sit in *vajrāsana* or any comfortable position. Raise your
arms in front and gently clench your fists with your
thumbs inside. Flick your fingers open and again clench.
Practise five to 10 times and then relax your arms.

Next clench your fists with the thumbs outside. Slowly
rotate your wrists clockwise and anticlockwise five to 10
times in each direction. Then relax your arms.

Raise your arms again and stretch your hands upward
and downward, bending from your wrists.

Be aware of all your hand muscle movements.

Now place your fingers on your shoulders and slowly
rotate your arms clockwise and anticlockwise five to 10
times in each direction. As you rotate your arms together,
exhale and when opening your arms, inhale. Be aware of
all your upper body muscle movements.

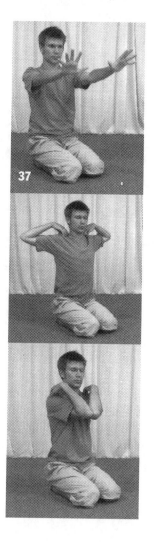

### 38. *Skandhayamasana* **shoulder blade stretch:**

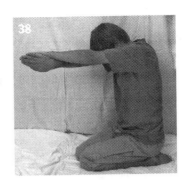

Continue sitting in *vajrasana* if you are comfortable. If not, come into a kneeling position. Raise your arms in front, shoulder height, cross your wrists and place your palms together.

Inhale slowly pulling your arms forward from your shoulders. Exhale while lowering your head forward. Remain in this position and breathe gently. Be aware of the stretch underneath your shoulder blades. While you are in this position, swap your hands over and notice if makes any difference to the stretch beneath your shoulder blades.

### 39. *Shankasthasana* **shellfish pose:**

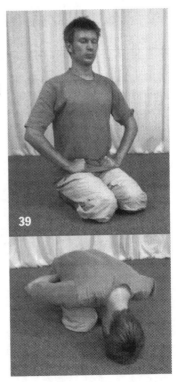

Sit in *vajrasana*. Place your palms on your thighs close to hips. Point your fingers inwards and then make fists so that your knuckles are pointing upwards.

Pull up from your lower back inhaling and slowly bend forward exhaling. Look to the front while bending forward. When you come half way, lower your head towards the floor. If you have high blood pressure keep your head up and do not bend so that your head is lower then your heart. As you roll forward be aware of your fists pressing into your ascending and descending colons. Remain there for a moment breathing gently. Then inhale slowly raising your head and slowly sit up. Repeat three or four times.

This *asana* enhances the digestive system and female reproductive system.

### 40. *Mandirasana* **temple pose:**

Sitting in *vajrasana*, place your palms on your thighs and inhale slowly while raising your arms above your head. Exhale placing your palms together and bending your elbows keeping your hands in a prayer position above your head. Gently pull your shoulder blades closer and be aware of your upper body.

Hold this *asana* breathing gently and then release after a few seconds. Immediately continue with the next *asana*.

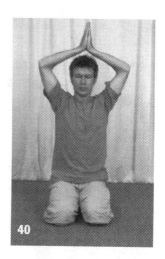

### 41. *Phani asana* **hooded snake pose:**

Kneel up onto your shins while inhaling slowly and straightening your arms above your head. The arms should now be in alignment with your shoulders. Slightly lean back by pushing your pelvis forward while exhaling. Be aware of the gentle bend in your back. Inhale straightening up. Exhale slowly sitting into *vajrasana* with your hands on your thighs. Again feel into your lower back. Repeat this combination of *mandirasana* and *phani asana* four to seven times and then relax into the next pose.

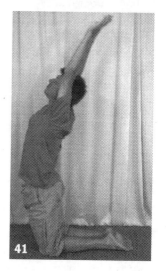

### 42. *Ushtrasana* **camel pose variation:**

DO NOT DROP YOUR HEAD BACKWARDS IF YOU HAVE A PROBLEM IN THE CERVICAL SPINE.

Kneel on your shins and place your hands on your rump area. This is the base position for this variation of *ushtrasana*.

Inhale slowly drawing your shoulder blades closer together then exhale gradually bending back and pushing your pelvis forward. Be aware of your back as you hold and also feel the stretch to the front of your torso. Inhale slowly returning to your base position. Practise this variation of *ushtrasana* two or three times.

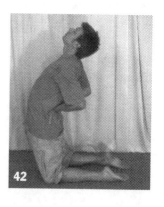

### 43. *Katayamasana* **hip stretching pose:**

From the kneeling position, bring your legs together and then lunge with your right foot in front. Place both of your hands on the floor inside of your right foot. Turn your left toes turned under so the ball of your foot is against the floor. Check that your right knee is not lunging further forward than your big toe. Now look at the floor.

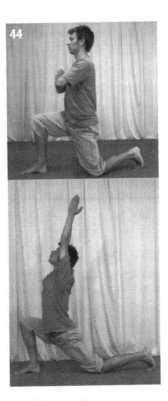

Inhale gently while lifting your left knee and pushing your lower back down. Be aware of the stretch in your left hip flexure muscles. Hold for a few seconds as you continue to breathe normally and then slowly release placing your left knee on the floor again. Practise this stretch two or three times and then prepare for *chandrodayasana* on the right side by resting your hands either side of your right foot.

### 44. *Chandroday-asana* **rising moon pose:**

The next *asana* is a combination of two postures. The first is *ashwa sanchalanasana* galloping horse pose followed by *ardha chandrasana* crescent moon pose.

From your lunging position with your hands placed either side of your right foot, check that your right knee is not lunging further forward than your big toe. Looking up, place your fingertips on the floor and slowly inhale. Hold this position for a moment and mentally locate your eyebrow center. Exhale slowly while relaxing your head forward and resting your palms on the floor. Now slowly inhale as you lift your torso and place your hands in a prayer position in front of your chest. Hold the prayer position and be aware of the centre of your chest.

Before moving into the next posture, exhale fully. As you commence inhalation, slowly start to stretch your arms above your head while keeping your palms

*44 continues next page*

together. In this position lean back slightly. Hold the pose and be aware of your lower back. Exhale while returning to a lunging position with your hands either side of your front foot. Practise this sequence three to five times. When you have finished, perform *katayamasana* on the left side followed by *chandrodayasana*.

### 45. *Indudalasana* **crescent moon pose:**

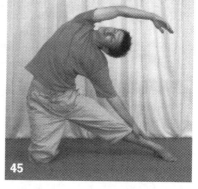

Kneel on your shins and stretch your right leg to the side, placing your foot in such a way that you can balance yourself. Rest your right hand on your right thigh, left arm relaxed by your side. Inhale slowly while lifting your left arm and turn the palm towards you. Exhale slowly bending right, allowing your right hand to slide down your right leg. Your left arm curls in a relaxed way over your head. Remain in the posture breathing gently and be aware of the compression in your right side and stretch through your left. Also feel the lateral stretch in your back and spine. Inhale slowly returning to your base position. Practise two or three times and then perform the *indudalasana* on the other side.

### 46. *Tad-asana* **palm tree pose:**

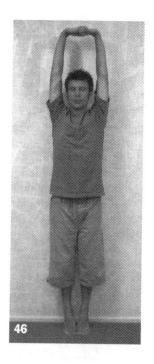

Stand for a few moments with your eyes closed and bring your awareness to your position. Check that your feet are parallel; your knees neither locked back nor bent; tuck your tailbone forward; lift your sternum and pull head back slightly. Open your eyes and prepare for *tadasana*. Keep your legs together, toes spread slightly, fingers interlaced and gazed fixed ahead. While inhaling slowly stretch your arms above your head, turn your palms upward and lift onto the balls of your feet. Remain in the pose while breathing gently.

Be aware of the stretch through your arms and torso, front and back. Feel your legs and feet balancing you. If you lose balance then tighten your buttocks and gently pull your abdominal muscles in. Release slowly while fully exhaling.

This *asana* assists lymphatic drainage in the armpits, stretches the vertebrae away from each other, strengthens the leg muscles and improves your physical and mental balance. Even if you do not have time to practise *yoga* each day at least do this one *asana*.

### 47. *Ashwatasana* holy fig tree pose:

This *asana* can be practiced during pregnancy as it improves foetal blood supply. Lift your right arm above your head with the palm facing the wall in front; lift your left arm shoulder height with your palm facing the floor. Take your left leg back, placing your big toe on the floor to maintain your balance. Gradually lift your left leg a few centimeters and hold this position up to 30 seconds while breathing gently.

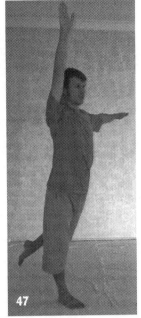

Be aware of your lower back while holding your position. Lower your leg first, then your arms and practise on the other side. This *asana* is particularly beneficial for the lower back.

### 48. *Dwikonasana* 2-angle pose:

Stand with your feet placed hip width apart. Interlace your fingers behind your back. Inhale and start to pull your shoulder blades together. Exhale while bending forward from your hips, lifting your arms as you bend. Keep looking to the front and when your torso is almost parallel to floor, then look towards the floor. Bend as far forward as comfortable while stretching your shoulders.

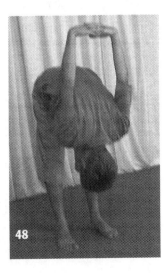

If you have high blood pressure do not lower your head below your heart. Breathe gently while you hold for a few seconds. Then start to relax your arms and raise your head while inhaling slowly and stand. Immediately continue with the next *asana*.

### 49. *Prishtayamasana* **back stretching pose:**

After *dwikonasana* exhale slowly while dropping your head back and bending backwards with bent knees.

Inhale slowly, lifting your head and pulling your shoulder blades together and continue with *dwikonasana*. Combine these two *asana* postures three or four times and then relax after the last forward bend.
**Stand for a few moments with your eyes closed and feel your body before continuing with the next *asana*.**

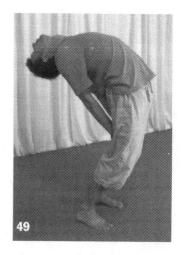

### 50. *Akarna dhanurasana*
**standing drawing the bow pose:**

Stand with your feet about one metre apart and look straight ahead. Turn your right foot away from you and then turn your body to face the wall on your right. Your left foot will be at a right angle to your body. Slide your left heel back a few centimeters. Make gentle fists and raise your arms shoulder height. The thumb part of your fist faces upward. Your right arm will extend further forward than your left. This is the base position for *akarna dhanurasana*.

As you inhale slowly draw your left fist back towards your left shoulder and extend your right arm further forward without leaning forward. Remain in this position and breathe gently. Be aware of all the areas of your body this posture affects. Release slowly while exhaling and return to the base position. Practise three to five times on this side. Then turn and practise on the other side.

Stand with your feet hip width apart and relax your arms beside you. Rotate your shoulders forward three times and then backwards three times.

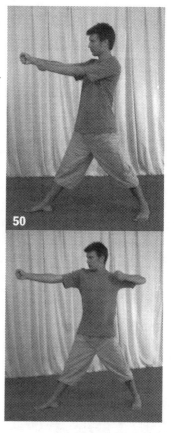

### 51. *Urayamasana* **chest stretch pose:**

Place your feet about one metre apart and feet straight ahead. Either hold your forearms behind your back or place your hands in prayer position. Keep your legs in the same base position as *akarna dhanur-asana,* right leg in front. Inhale gently pulling your shoulder blades closer. Exhale slowly bending your head backwards. Inhale lift your head and torso. Practise this *asana* two or three times.

Return to the central position. Slowly turn your fingers downwards from the prayer position and release. Raise your arms in front, level with your shoulders, and bend your hands upwards and downwards a few times. Make gentle fists and rotate your hands in one direction and then the other. Now practise *urayamasana* on the other side.

This *asana* affects all the areas of your upper body including thyroid gland.

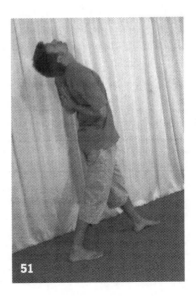

51

**52.** *Utthita mandirashira asana* **standing hamstring stretch:**

Stand in the same base position as *akarna dhanurasana* and turn towards your right. Relax your arms by your sides. Inhale raising your arms above your head.

Exhale slowly while bending your right knee and bending forward from your hips. Look to the front as you bend. When your torso is almost parallel to the floor lower your head and place your hands either side of your foot. Slowly straighten your right knee.

Remain in the pose for a few seconds while breathing gently. Be aware of your right hamstring stretching and relax into it. Release slowly inhaling and again bend your right knee; raise your head and lift your arms above your head as you stand up. Straighten your right knee and exhale lowering your arms. Turn to the central position and then practise on the other side. Practise once or twice on both sides.

**Walk your feet together until they are hip width apart. Stand with your eyes closed for a few moments being aware of your whole body.**

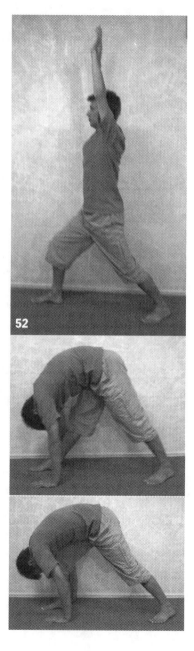

### 53. *Trikonasana* **triangle pose**

**Variation one:**
Stand in the same base position with your right foot turned towards the right. Keep your hips square to the front, arms relaxed by your sides. Inhale slowly raising your arms shoulder height, palms turned downwards. Exhale while lunging right. Be aware not to roll the arch of your right foot or drop your right knee inwards. As you lunge do not bend your knee further forward than your big toe. While exhaling take your right arm down the right leg and left arm straight up with your palm facing forward.

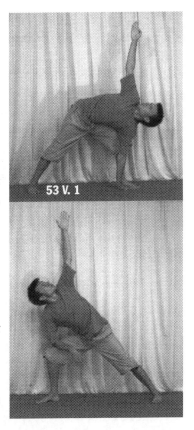

53 V. 1

You can place your right arm in various positions: bend your elbow and rest your forearm above your knee; or take your hand down to your ankle and hold; or place your palm on the floor outside of your foot; or place your palm on the floor inside of your foot. Look at your left arm and check that it is vertical. Look back to the centre. Feel the parts of your body you are working on. Hold for 10 to 20 seconds and then release or practise the second and third variations.

**Variation two:**
Slowly lower your left arm over your head so it is parallel to the floor.

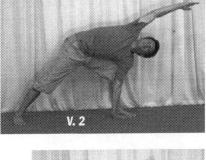

V. 2

**Variation three:**
When your right arm is vertical, turn your palm backwards, bend your elbow and place the back of your hand behind your back. Be aware of the areas of your body that are affected. Slowly release inhaling, raise your left arm and stand up with your arms stretched shoulder height. Exhale slowly while lowering your arms.

Continue *trikonasana* on the other side.

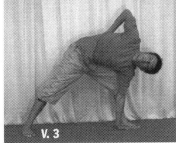

V. 3

*See next page for variation four*

### 53. *Trikon<u>a</u>sana* **triangle pose:** *(continued)*

**Variation four:**
Stand with your feet about one metre apart, feet placed at a 45-degree angle to your body. Inhale while lifting your arms shoulder height, palms turning downwards. Slowly exhale while bending forward and keeping your arms shoulder height. When your head is almost parallel straighten your neck. Remain in a position that creates a 90-degree angle between your back and legs.

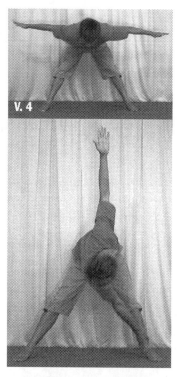

Take your right hand across to your left foot or shin. Your left arm should be vertical. Look up your left arm, palm turned to the front. Do not twist your forearm. Be aware of all the areas of your body affected by this *<u>a</u>sana*. Inhale back to the 90-degree angle, and perform on the other side. Practise on both sides two or three times. Then inhale slowly and return to the 90-degree angle and stand up with your arms raised shoulder height. Exhale while lowering your arms.

Apart from working on the spine, back, arm and leg muscles, this *<u>a</u>sana* also massages the digestive system, tones the reproductive area and nervous system.

### 54. *Utthita jang<u>a</u>yam<u>a</u>sana* **standing thigh stretch:**

Balance on your left foot and bend your right knee taking hold of your right foot with your right hand. Pull your heel into your buttock to stretch your thigh. Release the stretch and keep holding your foot. Raise your left arm above your head with the palm towards the wall in front.

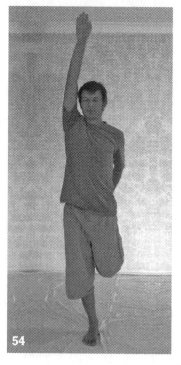

Inhale while stretching your left arm upward and pulling your heel into your buttock. Exhale slowly and release the position. Practise this *<u>a</u>sana* on the other side.

**55.** *Uttitha lolasana* **standing swing pose:**

This *asana* prepares you for *pranayama* breathing. Stand with your feet separated a little wider than your hips. Inhale slowly through your nose raising your arms above your head.

Flop forward from your hips while exhaling through your mouth and producing a haaaa sound. Hang in the position for a few moments breathing gently.

When you stand up, begin by first raising your head and then lift your arms while inhaling. Practise five to eight times.

If you have a back problem, bend your knees as you flop forward. If you have high blood pressure do not flop forward with your head lower than your heart.

**After practicing the standing *asana* postures you can perform *uddiyana bandha* standing and then lie down in *shavasana*. Alternatively, sit and develop body steadiness *kaya sthairyam*.**

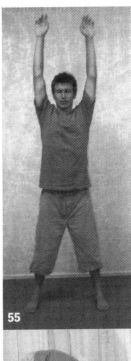

55

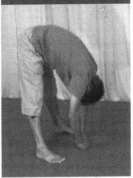

# CHAPTER FIVE

# *Pranayama:* Breath Utilisation

When the *prana* (vital energy) moves the *chitta* (mental content) will also move.
When the *prana* is without movement, the *chitta* is without movement.
By steadying the *prana*, the yogi attains steadiness and should therefore restrain the *vayu* (air).

*(Hatha Yoga Pradipika:* chapter 2 verse 2)

*Hatha yoga* teaches various techniques of breathing utilizing oxygen intake and carbon dioxide expulsion, ability to retain your breath in and out, as well as involving your nervous system, and right/left brain hemisphere activities. The *yogic* breathing techniques can be more powerful than the *asana* postures in terms of developing mental abilities and meditation. Breath is the link between mind and body, between your vital energy system and your body, and between your vital energy system and your mind.

The word *pranayama* is made up of two words *prana* and *ayama*. *Prana* literally means a force in motion and *ayam* means to stretch or expand. Through the techniques of *pranayama* you are con-

trolling your breath in order to expand your *prana* vital energy.

First of all, you need to become aware of the natural movement of your spontaneous breath. The diaphragm muscle between your lungs and rib cage initiates inhalation by contracting and pulling the ribs and lungs open, this sucks the air in through your nostrils. When you exhale the diaphragm muscle relaxes, pushing the ribs and lungs closed and expelling the air out of the nostrils. If the diaphragm muscle is traumatised then you cannot breath properly.

**Practice one:**

Lie on your back in *shavasana* relaxation pose. Place your hands on the stomach area above your navel, middle fingers tips in contact with each other. As you breath in spontaneously you will feel the hands lift and middle fingers moving away. As you exhale you will feel your hands dropping and middle finger tips moving back together again. When you practice *pranayama* breathing you do not change this natural rhythm. What will change is the depth of your breath, speed of your breath and whether you retain your breath or not.

**Practice two:**

Continue to lie in *shavasana* relaxation pose and place your hands on your abdomen below the navel and above the pubic bone. Take control of your breath and slowly inhale while consciously expanding the abdomen. Be aware of your hands lifting upward as the abdomen rises. And feel the pressure created within your abdomen. If you can, feel this movement pushing back into the lumbar and sacral spine. Then continue to exhale slowly with control, being aware of your abdomen relaxing down and the inner pressure releasing. Make sure your body is completely relaxed throughout this practice. The majority of movement is happening in your abdomen, while your stomach and chest areas are relaxed with minimal movement. Practise 10 to 15 breaths.

Next place your hands up to your stomach area, just above your navel. Inhale slowly, expanding and lifting your stomach area, while allowing your abdomen and chest to remain relaxed. Now you can feel the internal pressure in the stomach area and into the thoracic area of your spine. Exhale slowly feeling the pressure releasing. Practise 10 to 15 breaths.

Lastly place your hands beneath your collarbones, high up on the chest. Allow the abdomen and stomach area to be relaxed while inhaling slowing and lifting the chest area. Feel the pressure within your upper chest and through to the upper spine. Exhale slowly feeling the pressure releasing. Practise 10 to 15 breaths.

**Practice three:**

Lie in *shavasana*. Inhale gradually while first expanding your abdomen, then stomach area, then your chest. When you exhale first relax your the abdomen, then the stomach area and lastly your chest. During inhalation and exhalation both rotate your awareness first to your abdomen, then your stomach area and then your chest. While moving your abdomen count mentally one, two, three; while moving the stomach area, count four, five, six and seven at your chest. Practise for a few minutes.

**Practice four:**

Continue lying in *shavasana*. During abdominal breathing visualize or imagine that you are inhaling through the soles of your feet and the air ascends to your head. As you exhale the air descends back down and is expelled through the soles of your feet.

**Stage two:** Develop this visualization further. While practising abdominal breathing, imagine your inner body is hollow and your skin is the shell of your body. Create an idea that you are inhaling the earth's energy through the soles of your feet. Imagine this energy permeating your body as it ascends to the crown of your head. During exhalation imagine the air only descending and arouse a feeling of letting go of resistance. As you breath out through the soles of your feet release all tiredness, tension and negative impressions.

**Stage three:** Inhale the earth's energy up through the soles of your feet to the crown of your head, whilst being aware of the energy permeating the body internally. Retain the breath for a moment and imagine a sphere of rainbow light at the crown of your head. Slowly exhale, allowing the rainbow light to cascade down through each part of your body to your feet. This can later be practised with *ujjayi pranayama* as described below.

## *Nadi shodhana pranayama*
### alternate nostril breathing:

*Nadi shodhan* literally means purification of the energy pathways, referring to *ida*, *pingala* and *sushumna*. Sit in a comfortable position either on the floor or in a chair with your spine upright. Place your hands on your thighs or knees, center your head, lift your chest and slightly draw your head backwards. If possible, use your right hand to alternate the flow of breath in your nostrils because energy flows in through your left hand and out your right hand. By resting your right index and middle fingers at your eyebrow centre you are creating an energy circuit.

Close your right nostril with your thumb and slowly inhale through your left nostril. Close your left nostril with your ring finger. Release the right nostril and exhale slowly. Again breathe in through

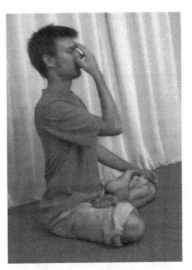

your right nostril and then close it, exhale through your left nostril. This is one round. During this round you may have become aware of a blockage in airflow in either nostril.

**Stage one:** While inhaling left mentally count- one, two, three, exhale right one, two, three; inhale right one, two, three, exhale left one, two, three. When inhalation and exhalation are equal, the ratio is called 1:1. Gradually you can extend the length of your breath by counting up to four, five, six, etc.

Make sure you do not inhale more than you exhale otherwise you will feel light headed or dizzy. This is an indication that you are hyperventilating. To rectify this, cup your hands over your nose and breathe normally until the dizziness ceases. Once you are proficient counting your breath, then you can include another concept. During inhalation imagine your breath ascending through your nostril to your eyebrow centre and descending through your nostril during exhalation. Practise 10 to 20 rounds in one sitting. When you feel proficient with this stage continue to next step.

**Stage two:** Practise step one and include breath retention after inhaling by closing both nostrils with your thumb and ring finger. While holding your breath, imagine the breath remaining at the eyebrow centre and count the same count as inhalation and exhalation. Now your ratio is 1:1:1, i.e. breathing in one, two, three; holding one, two, three; exhaling one two, three. Practise 10 to 20 rounds in one sitting. When you feel proficient with this stage continue to next step.

**Stage three:** Continue with same process as step two and now double your exhalation so the ratio becomes 1:1:2, i.e. breathing in three counts, holding three counts, exhaling six counts. Practise 10 to 20 rounds in one sitting. When you

feel proficient with this stage continue to next step.

**Stage four:** Continue step three and include external breath retention. Once you have exhaled retain your breath out by closing both nostrils and hold for the same duration as inhalation. Your ratio is now 1:1:2:1. Practise 10 to 20 rounds in one sitting. When you feel proficient with this stage continue to next step.

**Stage five:** Increase your ratio to 1:2:2:1 so that you now inhale for three counts, hold for six counts, exhale for six counts and hold again for three counts. Practise 10 to 20 rounds in one sitting.

## *Ujjayi pranayama* **stabilizing breathe:**

*Ujjayi* literally means victorious. As you practise *asana* regularly, over a period of time *ujjayi pranayama* happens spontaneously. It has a calming and centring affect on the mind and body and is therefore useful to regulate high blood pressure. *Ujjayi pranayama* is also an essential practice of specific meditation techniques.

**Stage one:** *Ujjayi* breathing is slow and controlled. This practice produces a soft sound from the flow of air passing in your throat. The sound should not be made in your voice box. To hear this sound, first of all breathe out through your mouth as if you are going to clean a smudge off glass. Listen to the *haaa* sound as you exhale. Then inhale in the same way as if you are gasping. Now listen to the *aahhh* sound.

*Ujjayi pranayama* is practised with the mouth closed. Exhale keeping your lips together and imagine you are breathing out onto your teeth. The sound will be a lot softer with your mouth closed. Inhale as if you are gasping. Breathe slowly and listen to the gentle sound of your breath *aahhhh haaaaa.* If you can't hear the sound properly, close one ear for a few moments and the sound will be more audible.

*Ujjayi pranayama* can be practised while performing *asana*, *mudra* or meditation, sitting, standing or lying down. You can even do it sitting on the bus to calm your mind before and after work.

## Swara yoga

According to the tantric tradition of **Swara yoga**, it is important to be aware of the significance of breathing through your right, left and both nostrils. To distinguish whether the volume of air is greater in either nostril, breathe out with a little force onto your fingertips. A more forceful flow in your right nostril indicates that the **surya** sun *swara* and the *pingala nadi* (positively charged energy) are active. When your breath is stronger in your left nostril then your **chandra** moon *swara* or *ida nadi* (negatively charged energy) are flowing. Sometimes your breath will feel perfectly even in both nostrils. This indicates the flow of the **shunya** void *swara* through *sushumna nadi*. *Sushumna* is the pathway through which the energy of spirit/soul/consciousness **atma shakti** flows. In the practice of *Swara yoga* it is necessary to

intimately understand these three types of *swara*, i.e. *surya*, *chandra* and *shunya*.

Try to evaluate your breath during sunrise because your *swara* usually synchronizes with the moon phase at this time. By checking your *swara* you will become more aware of your physical and mental rhythms throughout the day and night. When you wake up, touch your face on the same side as the active *swara* and step onto the floor with the same foot corresponding to the active *swara*. This ritual will remind you of your active energy flow and prevent you from 'getting out of bed on the wrong side'!

Ancient *tantrik* practitioners observed that the breath flows predominantly in the right nostril at sunrise on the first, second and third lunar dates, **titthi**, of the dark fortnight **krishna paksha**, i.e. the waning moon phase. Throughout the day the breath changes over from the right to left nostril and continues to alternate during 24 hours depending on the activities undertaken, diet, general state of health and weather. For the next three *titthi* lunar dates, fourth, fifth and sixth, the left nostril flows predominantly at sunrise, then from the seventh, eighth and ninth the left flows, from the tenth, eleventh and twelfth the right, and thirteenth, fourteenth and fifteenth the left. The breath then continues to alternate at sunrise on every third *titthi* lunar date during the bright fortnight **shukla paksha**, i.e. the waxing moon phase.

The most accurate time to evaluate your *swara* is at the confluence of night and day because your body is finishing its period of rest and starting to wake. There are less disturbing influences on the breath when you lie still during the night. The breath can also be checked at sunset, however, this time can be unsuitable if you live a hectic lifestyle. In *Swara yoga* the periods when day meets night or night meets day, are called **sandhya**. It is also a time of energetic changeover. The most significant *sandhya* is internal, when the mental and physical energies merge in the eyebrow centre. This is the time when a meditative experience is likely to unfold.

Back in the 1970's science discovered that 'every 90 minutes there is a brain storm'*, that every hour and a half the predominant brain energies move from one brain hemisphere to the other. In terms of *Swara yoga*, the faculties of *ida* and left nostril breathing correlate to right-brain hemisphere activities; *pingala* and right nostril breathing correlate with left-brain hemisphere activities. When the *chandra* lunar *swara* in the left nostril is active then quiet, passive, introverted or creative activities should be undertaken; while dynamic and practical activities are conducive during the *surya* solar *swara* in the right nostril. Each *swara* flows for an hour or more and then changes over. During the change over period the breath flows evenly in both nostrils, *shunya swara*. This is a time when the mental and physical energies are balanced, when the mind is neither extroverted nor introverted. It is also associated with activity in the corpus callosum. By practising *yoga* you balance *ida* and *pingala* and promote an even flow of air in your nostrils to encourage spontaneous meditation. Activities conducted in the external world when your *shunya swara* is active, usually do not prosper.

If you notice a persistent flow in one *swara* for several days, or if there is an overall predominant *swara* flow on a permanent basis, this reflects an imbalance of your inner state of being. For example you may observe that your left nostril functions more often than your right, which means the body's cooling system is over active and the heating system suppressed. It indicates problems such as sluggish digestion, cough, cold, lethargy, depression or even excessive psychic energy. Likewise overactivity of the body's heating system due to excessive breathing in your right nostril can result in fever, anxiety, excessive bowel motions or insomnia, just to mention a few conditions. One of the main reasons you practice the various *Hatha yoga* techniques is to maintain a balance between your physical heating/cooling systems and physical/mental energies. You can make a daily diary of your *swara* to see the effects of *ida*, *pingala* and *sushumna*. Make a note of your *swara* at sunrise and at the end of the day record the events and how you dealt with them.

*Psychology Today Nov. 1979 M. H. Chase*

*Swara yoga* also explains that each specific day of the week is influenced predominantly by either the feminine *ida* principle or the masculine *pingala* principle. You can achieve optimum results in your work and business while acting according to this principle *swara* energy of the day. For example, for business dealings, applying for a bank loan, buying a house or going for a job interview, your desired results can be achieved during the following times:

with your hands. When the breath flows out from the middle of your nostrils it reflects the presence of *prithvi* earth element, the flow from the bottom outer side of the nostril is *apas* water element, an upward flow towards the top rim of the nostril is *agni* fire element and *vayu* air element flows from the outer middle edge of the nostril. When the breath is very gentle, flowing all around and you can't discern the angle, it is *akasha* ether element.

| Day | | Optimum Time During | Moon phase |
|---|---|---|---|
| Sunday - | SUNday | Right *surya swara* | waning |
| Monday - | MOONday | Left *chandra swara* | waxing |
| Tuesday - | MARSday | Right *surya swara* | waning |
| Wednesday - | MERCURYday | Left *chandra swara* | waxing |
| Thursday - | JUPITERday | Left *chandra swara* | waxing |
| Friday - | VENUSday | Left *chandra swara* | waxing |
| Saturday - | SATURNday | Right *surya swara* | waning |

When life doesn't unfold quite as you plan, it reflects in your *swara* as an imbalance of your personal energy in relation to your environment.

The next stage in *Swara yoga* is to determine the angle at which your breath flows out from your nostril. The specific angle denotes an inherent *tattwa* element activity. Feel the angle of your breath

In the practice of *Swara yoga* you perform *shanmukhi mudra*, closing the upper gates of perception, to perceive the active *tattwa*. Press your ears with your thumbs, the eyelids with your index fingers, your nostrils with your middle fingers and lips with your ring and little fingers above and below. Hold *shanmukhi mudra* with internal or external breath retention while looking into *chi-*

*dakasha*, the back of your eyelids. When earth element is present you can see the color yellow and the shape of a square; water, a white crescent moon; fire, a red inverted triangle; air, a blue-grey hexagon and ether a circular non specific coloured form; ether contains all colours. Charts of the *tattwa* forms can be made for *trataka*, open-eyed meditation, to improve your power of visualization. Gaze at each form externally and then hold *shanmukhi mudra* watching whatever appears in *chidakasha*.

How do you interpret the *tattwa* elemental energies in your daily life? Think about the physical nature of the element itself to have a better understanding. Earth represents solidity and stability, so when the earth element is present in your breath it is displaying these qualities within yourself and what you will attract. Therefore it is a suitable time for actions requiring a stable outcome, e.g., purchasing your permanent place of residence. Water element is similar to earth, however it is not as stable. Water represents fluctuations and change after a period of time. Fire is the exact opposite. Just as fire burns and transmutes, so does the fire element. When you notice the fire element in your breath it alerts you to change, excitement, anger, even harm. Air element too represents instability. Just as air itself moves constantly and is erratic, so the air element in your breath indicates a time of uncertainty. Ether element is the most illusive of all and is of no consequence in your daily life, its only purpose is for meditation.

The most common question to arise when learning about *Swara yoga* is whether you can change the flow of your *swara* if needed? In some cases it is appropriate to adjust your breathing pattern. If you suffer insomnia, most likely you breathe predominantly through your right nostril. Therefore lie on your right side so the left nostril is uppermost and eventually you will drift off to sleep. Alternatively, you can rub the joining area of your thumb and index finger on the same side as the blocked *swara* to assist the airflow on that side. If that does not work, you could plug an incessantly flowing nostril with a small ball of cotton wool. However, a chronic obstruction caused by a deviated septum would need an operation to rectify the problem. Other obstructions such as polyps can be removed by practising *jala neti* nasal irrigation.

There are occasions, however, when the most appropriate course of action is simply to be in the state of *sakshi bhava* witnessing objectively. The knowledge of *swara* will help you realize that you may be able control your mind, your emotions, your psyche, your energies, your actions but some events happen beyond your anticipation and the best action is to surrender to the higher force.

# CHAPTER SIX

# Muscle Squeezing: *Bandha*

*Contracting the perineum, (mula bandha), practising uddiyana (bandha), ida and pingala are bound together and the air moves in the spinal passage (sushumna).*

(*Hatha Yoga Pradipika:* chapter 3 verse 75)

*Bandha* is a process of contracting specific muscle groups together to fetter the various energy flows. Traditionally *Hatha yoga* is practised in the sequence of *asana*, then *pranayama*, followed by *mudra* and lastly *bandha*. Quite often *pranayama, mudra* and *bandha* are combined together.

### *Jalandhara bandha* throat lock:

DO NOT PRACTISE JALANDHARA BANDHA IF YOU HAVE HIGH BLOOD PRESSURE.
Sit cross-legged or sit in a chair resting your hands on your knees. Inhale slowly then retain your breath. Lift your shoulders and lean forward pushing against your knees. Bend your head forward and remain in this position as long as possible.

Before you need to breathe, raise your head, drop your shoulders and then exhale slowly with your head upright. You can also practise in the same way while holding external breath retention.

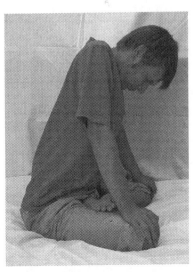

### *Uddiyana bandha* **stomach lock:**

DO NOT PRACTISE *UDDIYANA BANDHA* IF YOU
HAVE STOMACH ULCER, HERNIA OR HIGH
BLOOD PRESSURE.

Stand with your feet hip width apart,
bend your legs and place your hands
above your knees. Keep your head up
while inhaling fully, exhale through
your mouth, retain your breath out
and come into *jalandhara bandha*.
Gently draw your stomach inwards
and upwards.

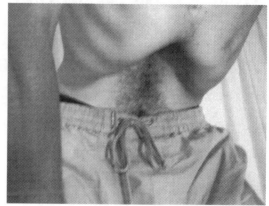

Hold as long as comfortable. Before
inhaling, relax your stomach, raise
your head and stand upright, then
slowly breath in.

Once you have perfected this *bandha* in a standing
position you can commence in a sitting position. If
you need to sit in a chair, then separate your legs and
place your hands on your knees. Exhale fully and lean
forward practising *jalandhara bandha* holding external
breath retention. Pull your stomach in and up slightly.
Release by relaxing your stomach, raising your head
and sitting upright, then inhale. Do not breathe while
lifting or lowering your head, only once you are upright
otherwise you can strain your neck muscles. Practise up
to five times on an empty stomach, preferably in the
morning.

*Uddiyana bandha* tones your internal organs and
muscles. It also strengthens your solar plexus region,
which in turn affects your emotional responses to life.

### *Nauli karma* **churning the rectus abdominus muscles:**

Perform *uddiyana bandha* from a standing position. Lift your right hand a centimeter and the rectus abdominus muscles will move left. Replace your hand and lift your left hand a centimeter. The rectus abdominus muscles will move right. Replace your hand and continue alternating a few more times. Relax your stomach and release *uddiyana bandha*. As you practise in this way you will gain control of your rectus abdominus muscles. Once you gain control you will be able to pull your muscles right and left and hold in the middle at will.

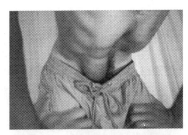
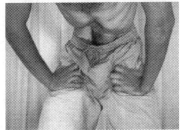
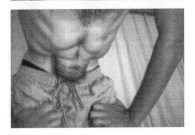

### *Mula bandha* **perineal lock:**

Sit in a comfortable position, take your awareness to the end of your spine then slowly pull your pelvic floor muscles up towards the spine base. As you become more proficient you need to draw up specific muscles rather than all the muscles of the pelvic floor. In the male body you focus on contracting the perineal muscles, ***puling mula bandha***. In the female body you focus on contracting the muscles around your cervix, ***striling mula bandha***. Initially all the pelvic floor muscles will contract. As you practise *mula bandha* you will gradually learn to isolate the different muscles. The practice of *mula bandha* can assist you to control your nervous system and is therefore useful for nervous disorders, depleted energy and lack of or poor orgasm. During sexual intercourse impulses can be improved and prolonged by practising *mula bandha*.

### *Maha bandha* **great lock:**

Can be practised sitting on the floor with your legs crossed or straight in front. If you are unable to sit on the floor, sit in a chair with your legs hip width apart and hands on your thighs. First perform *jalandhara bandha*, then *uddiyana* and lastly *mula bandha*.

*great lock continues next page*

Release *mula bandha, uddiyana* and *jalandhara*.
If your legs are straight, have your hands on your
thighs; inhale, exhale, retain your breath out; slide
your hands to your shins coming into *jalandhara*,
then *uddiyana*, lastly *mula bandha*. Release *mula
bandha, uddiyana* and *jalandhara*, then sit up, sliding your hands to your thighs and inhale slowly.

Practise up to five times on an empty stomach.

*Maha bandha* is so called because you receive the
benefits of all three *bandha* practices.

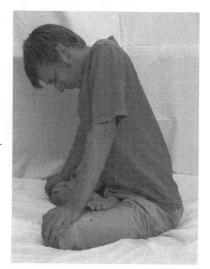

# CHAPTER SEVEN

# Energy Gestures: *Mudra*

*Therefore the goddess sleeping at
the Creator's entrance door should be constantly
aroused with all effort by performing mudra
thoroughly.*

(*Hatha Yoga Pradipika*: chapter 3 verse 5)

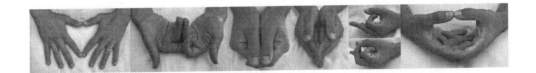

The sleeping goddess referred to in the *Hatha Yoga Pradipika* is the *kundalini* energy that can be aroused by the practising *mudra*. *Mudra* gesture is the physical expression of an inner attitude. It may occur spontaneously as you practise *yoga* daily, or you can employ known *mudra* gestures to achieve a desired outcome.

The *chakra mudra* gestures elucidated here enable you to consciously contact each *chakra* energy center. The process of *chakra shuddhi* combined with *mudra* assists the purification of each centre. *Mudra* can be practiced after *pranayama* or prior to meditation. It can be useful to keep a diary of your experiences after looking into *chidakasha*, as well as noting daily experiences and your dreams.

**1.** *Agya mudra* **gesture:**

Join your right thumb and index finger tips together and do the same with the left. Place both middle finger tips together, ring finger tips together and little finger tips together. The middle, ring and little fingers should point upward.

Fix your awareness in the centre of your head and repeat the *bija* mantra *Aum* either verbally or mentally.

## *Agya chakra mudra shuddhi* **purification:**

**Step one:** Hold *agya mudra* at the eyebrow centre *bhru madhya*. Imagine a point of white light in the centre of your head. Breathe in through the eyebrow centre to the point of white light and out the same way. Practise as long as you can hold *agya mudra* comfortably.

**Step two:** Incorporate *ujjayi pranayama*, inhale to the point of white light and as your breath reaches the white light imagine the light expanding, as you exhale out from *bhru madhya* the light contracts.

**Step three:** Watch the space in front of your closed eyes when you have finished. Observe your thoughts.

### 2. *Muladhara mudra* **gesture:**

Interlace your fingers, palms turned upward, thumbs tips joined; then point your middle fingers downward while joining them at the first phalange.

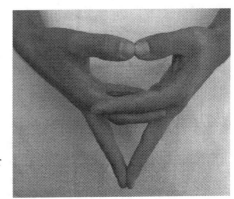

Fix your awareness below your tailbone and repeat the *bija* mantra *Lam* either verbally or mentally.

### *Muladhara chakra mudra shuddhi* **purification:**

**Step one:** Hold *muladhara mudra* in your lap; imagine a point of crimson light at *muladhara*. Create the idea of inhaling into the point of crimson light and exhaling out of the point.

**Step two:** Incorporate *ujjayi pranayama* with step one and imagine the crimson light expanding as you inhale and contracting as you exhale.

**Step three:** Watch the space in front of your closed eyes when you have finished. Observe your thoughts.

### 3 a. *Stri swadhisthana mudra* **female swadhisthana gesture:**

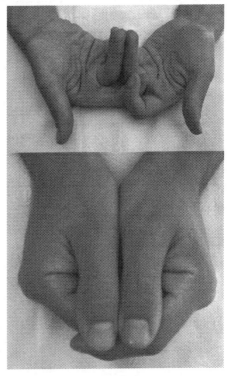

Interlace your fingers, palms facing upward, then slide your middle fingers inward placing the second phalange back to back. Now place your index fingers one on top of the other and rest your thumbs side by side at the first phalange.

Fix your awareness at your spine parallel to your pubic bone and repeat the *bija* mantra *Vam* either verbally or mentally.

### 3 b. *Vira swadhisthana mudra* **male** *swadhisthana* **gesture:**

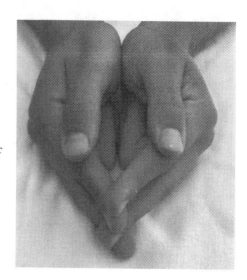

Interlace your middle and index fingers at the first phalange and point them downwards, turn your ring and little fingers in towards the palms and rest the back of the second phalanges together, keep the heels of your hands together and rest your thumbs against the third phalange of your index fingers.

Fix your awareness at your spine parallel to your pubic bone and repeat the *bija* mantra *Vam* either verbally or mentally.

### *Stri swadhisthana chakra mudra shuddhi* and *Vira swadhisthana chakra mudra* **purification:**

**Step one:** Hold *swadhisthana mudra* in your lap; imagine a point of vermilion light at *swadhisthana*. Create the idea of inhaling into the point of vermilion light and exhaling out of the point.

**Step two:** Incorporate *ujjayi pranayama* with step one and imagine the vermilion light expanding as you inhale and contracting as you exhale.

**Step three:** Watch the space in front of your closed eyes when you have finished. Observe your thoughts.

### 4. *Manipura mudra* **gesture:**

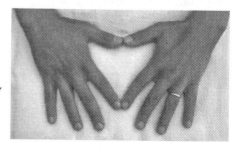

Join your thumb tips together, pointing them upward. Join your index finger tips pointing them downward.

The remaining fingers are spread comfortably apart.

Fix your awareness at your spine parallel to your navel and repeat the *bija* mantra *Ram* either verbally or mentally.

## *Manipura chakra shuddhi* **purification:**

**Step one:** Hold *manipura mudra* around your navel with your thumbs pointing towards your chest. Now imagine a golden star of light at *manipura*. Create an idea that you are breathing into this star when you inhale and breathing out from the star as you exhale.

**Step two:** Incorporate *ujjayi pranayama* with step one and imagine the golden star expanding when you inhale and contracting as you exhale.

**Step three:** Watch the space in front of your closed eyes when you have finished practicing steps one and two. Observe any thoughts that come into your mind.

## 5. *Anahata mudra* **gesture:**

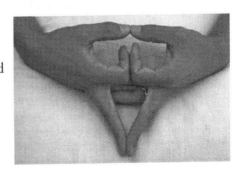

Interlace your fingers with the palms facing up; straighten your middle fingers downward so they join at tips; pull your index fingers up so they are back to back at the second phalange; place your thumbs upward so the tips join.

Fix your awareness at your spine between your shoulder blades and repeat the *bija* mantra *Yam* either verbally or mentally.

## *Anahata chakra mudra shuddhi* **purification:**

**Step one:** Hold *anahata mudra* in front of your sternum region and imagine a point of pale blue or pale pink light at *anahata*. Create the idea of inhaling into the point of pale blue or pale pink light and exhaling out from the point.

**Step two:** Incorporate *ujjayi pranayama* with step one and imagine the pale blue or pale pink light expanding as you inhale and contracting as you exhale.

**Step three:** Watch the space in front of your closed eyes when you have finished. Observe your thoughts.

### 6. *Vishuddhi mudra* **gesture:**

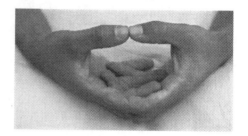

Interlace your fingers inwards, palms facing upward and thumb tips joined.

Fix your awareness at your spine in the center of your neck and repeat the *bija* mantra *Ham* either verbally or mentally.

### *Vishuddhi chakra mudra shuddhi* **purification:**

**Step one:** Hold *vishuddhi mudra* in front of your throat and imagine a point of purple light at *vishuddhi*. Create the idea of inhaling into the point of purple light and exhaling out of the point.

**Step two:** Incorporate *ujjayi pranayama* with step one and imagine the purple light expanding as you inhale and contracting as you exhale.

**Step three:** Watch the space in front of your closed eyes when you have finished. Observe your thoughts.

### 7. *Chin mudra* **gesture of the consciousness:**

Join your index fingers to the root of your thumbs, palms facing upward.

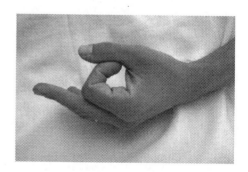

This *mudra* is used during the practice of meditation.

### 8. *Hridaya mudra* **gesture of the heart:**

Place your fingers in *chin mudra* and then join your middle and ring finger tips to your thumb tip.

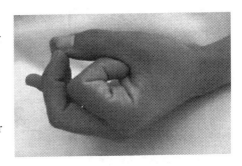

This *mudra* is also used during the practice of meditation. As it affects the cardiac plexus area and heart region, do not hold for extended periods of time.

### 9. *Khechari mudra* **gesture of one who flies in space:**

Curl your tongue back so the tip rests against the top palate. If you can, push the tip of your tongue further back against the soft palate. Keeping your tongue in this position may produce excess saliva so you will need to release it occasionally and swallow. Bitter tasting saliva indicates there are toxins in your body. However, during profound meditation the taste of saliva becomes sweet.

### 10. *Oli mudra* gesture is the process of sublimating sexual energy into *ojas* vital energy and strength. Because of the different reproductive systems in the male and female bodies the technique of *oli* is known by different names. **Sahajoli** is the practice for women and **vajroli** is for men. Essentially *sahajoli* and *vajroli* are the same practice. *Sahaj* literally means innate and *vajra* in this context means impenetrable.

### 10 a. *Sahajoli mudra* **for women:**

Gently tighten your urinary muscles inwards, as if you are stopping yourself from urinating. Women will feel a sensation in the labia with the action of *sahajoli mudra*. You should not practise if you have a urinary tract infection. *Sahajoli* can assist with incontinence and improve sexual function. It can be practised anytime as well as during intercourse to improve orgasm.

**10 b.** *Vajroli Mudra* **for men:**

Tighten your urinary muscles inwards as if you are stopping yourself from urinating. The testes will move a little with the action of *vajroli mudra*. Do not practise if you have a urinary tract infection. *Vajroli mudra* can assist with incontinence and improve sexual function. It can be practised anytime as well as during intercourse.

**11.** *Ashwini mudra* **horse gesture:**

Tighten the anal sphincter muscles inward as if you are stopping yourself from passing wind. If you have anal fistula then you should not practise *ashwini mudra*.

**12.** *Shambhavi mudra* **feminine energy gesture:**

Take your gaze upward without moving your head and look in towards your eyebrow center.

Hold as long as comfortable and then rest your eyes.

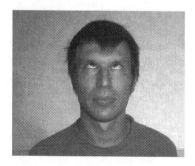

### 13. *Maha mudra* **great gesture:**

Sit cross-legged on a folded blanket or in a chair, with your spine upright, hands on your knees and tongue in *khechari mudra*. Inhale using *ujjayi* breathing, retain your breath inside and slightly tilt your head backward. Look up into your eyebrow center, *shambhavi mudra* and practise *mula bandha*.

While retaining your breath rotate your awareness, mentally repeating, *agya, vishuddhi, muladhara; agya, vishuddhi, muladhara; agya, vishuddhi, muladhara*, as long as you can hold comfortably. Release *shambhavi mudra* first, then *mula bandha*, straighten your head and exhale slowly with *ujjayi* breathing maintaining *khechari mudra*.

Remember, if you have high blood pressure or a heart condition then do not retain your breath inside. Or if you cannot hold your breath for any other reason, breathe gently while rotating your awareness *agya, vishuddhi, muladhara*.

### 14. *Shanmukhi mudra* **gesture of closing 7 openings:**

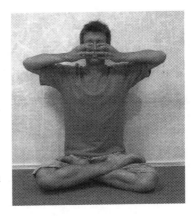

Sit in a comfortable position with your spine upright. Close your ears with your thumb tips and your index fingers resting on the edge of your closed eyelids. Place your middle fingers close to your nostrils but do not block your nose yet. Then rest your ring fingers above the upper lip and little fingers below the lower lip. Inhale slowly, retain your breath and close your nostrils.

If you have high blood pressure or heart condition do not close your nose or hold your breath, continue to breathe gently. Watch the space in front of your closed eyes *chidakasha*. To exhale, release your middle fingers from your nostrils and exhale slowly.

### 15. *Prana mudra* **energy flow gesture:**

Sit comfortably and place your hands in front of your abdomen, palms facing your body. Inhale and exhale slowly with *ujjayi*, retain your breath out and perform *mula bandha* continue to breathe gently if you have high blood pressure or heart disease. Release *mula bandha*.

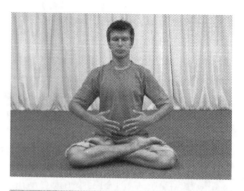

Inhale with *ujjayi*, simultaneously lifting your hands in front of your body and imagine that energy is ascending within your body in synchronisation with your hands and breath.

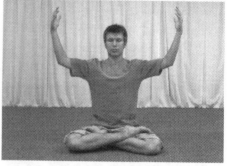

As your hands reach your face expand them sideways, level with your shoulder, palms turned upward and imagine the energy now expanding outward, like a flower blooming. While expanding your arms retain your breath. Continue to breathe gently if you have high blood pressure or heart disease.

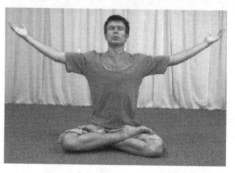

Exhale slowly with *ujjayi* and draw the energy back down into the abdominal cavity. Practise for a minute or two and then sit watching *chidakasha*.

# CHAPTER EIGHT

# Mind Absorption: Meditation

*I am the moon*
*You are the sun*
*Your light reflects off me*
*We are two and yet one*

(Muktibodha)

Meditation is a spontaneous function of the body and mind. Just as sleep occurs naturally without force, so it is with meditation. Sleep takes place when your body is still and your eyes are closed, then the mind introverts and drifts off. For meditation to occur your body also needs to become quiet first. Meditation is as much a function of your body as it is an experience in your mind. Yoga practices play an important role to balance the chemical structure of your body in preparation for meditation. When your body is tense, stressed, stiff, full of toxic chemicals, the process of meditation is difficult if not impossible. Regularity of your yoga practice and a balanced diet allows meditation to unfold more quickly.

The Sanskrit word for meditation, *dhyana*, implies a concentrated pattern of consciousness that is absorbed in the object of concentration. *Dhyana* occurs when you are continually absorbed in the perception of a particular form, or a sound, or picture or idea. During *dhyana* whatever occurs in the external physical world cannot affect your consciousness because you are observing yourself in the subconscious state. During meditation and subconscious dream state there is awareness of individuality; however, meditation is distinguished by the ability to observe yourself in this state. When a dream occurs you are aware of yourself in some form in the dream, even if you do not actually see yourself in the dream or know that you are dreaming. By developing the ability to know that you are in the dream state and can control your dream, then you are empowering your ability to meditate.

Meditation cannot occur by forcing or controlling your mind. It is as useless as lying in bed and saying, "I must sleep now, I am not asleep yet but I have to sleep immediately". It requires much patience and practice and the ability to observe yourself at every waking and meditating moment.

In India's history, **brahman** priests prepared certain herbs to induce transcendence. This was known as **aushadhi**. Today *aushadhi* refers to the use of herbs as medicine. A particular plant called **soma lata**, the golden creeper, was highly regarded by the *brahmans* to take them into a transcendental state. The **kshatriya** caste of kings and armies demanded the right to use it and unfortunately that sent them mad. So the *brahmans* decided to eradicate the *soma lata* vine.

Though the *soma* vine is not available in India, there are particular herbs in South America that some shamans can prepare to produce a similar effect. The specific preparation of ayahusca contains a chemical also produced by the brain itself. Taking ayahusca creates a profound state where all your problems can be answered, if you can understand the significance of what you see in the few minutes that the experience lasts. This may be a more effortless technique than practicing meditation but the side effects are more dangerous. Therefore, the use of ayahusca should be restricted to the guidance of a seasoned shaman.

Throughout history people have strived to attain transcendence or God consciousness. Very few have achieved it. However, with the natural evolution of the human brain, more people will experience deep states of meditation with less effort. You can choose to accelerate your process of evolution by practising *yoga* and meditation.

## The Practice

The various meditation techniques you learn today from your teacher or book are simply methods to induce meditation. When practising it is important not to control your mind. Rather be aware of whatever happens; allow your thoughts to come and go and observe like watching traffic pass; without judging whether it is a good or a bad thought, observe it as a mere thought. If you allow your mind to be free and to become still by itself then you are not antagonizing, suppressing or repressing your mind, rather you are accepting it. You have to understand that meditation is a state of awareness beyond mundane thoughts. In order to move beyond the casual thoughts you need to accept your state of mind and not fight it. You cannot achieve a true state of meditation when you are anxious, stressed or frustrated because you are caught in the reality of the external world. However, by employing the techniques of meditation you can reduce your reactions to the external stimulus.

The *Amritabindu Upanishad* text describes *that mind is the cause of bondage and liberation. The mind that is attached to material objects leads to bondage, while if it is dissociated from material objects it can lead to liberation.* Therefore you need to become aware of the nature of your mind and to realize there is something separate from your mind within you. In order to develop awareness of your mind take time out on your own and watch yourself objectively.

Practising meditation should be effortless. If the traditional system of performing *asana, pranayama, mudra, bandha* or employing *yama*, and *niyama* is not possible then try lying in bed before sleeping or just after waking and focus on your breath. Weave your meditation into your daily routine so it becomes a facet of your life.

Traditionally meditation is practised sitting on the floor. However, you may choose to sit in a chair or lie in *shavasana*. Whatever your position, as far as possible, keep your spine in alignment so the nervous impulses and energy can run freely between your body and brain.

## Chetana Jagriti

The basis of all *yoga* practice is the ability to witness yourself, known as *sakhshi bhava*. Literally *sakshi bhava* means the feeling of being a witnesser. As discussed our mind and body are the aggregate of many different aspects and elements. By enabling part of your mind to stand back and observe the various aspects of yourself you are awakening your consciousness, **chetana jagriti**.

Start by observing yourself in any situation. Be aware that part of your mind is standing back objectively watching you in your current environment. When you watch a film you are the observer of that film. In the same way watch yourself in the film of life! You are the silent onlooker of all the other aspects of your mind and body and whatever you are doing. Be the witness of all your movements, walking, standing, sitting, breathing….

Be the witnesser of the different sounds you hear close by, distant…..

When you talk listen to yourself while you are talking, watch yourself listening to the other person. Watch the thoughts that arise while you are talking, while you are listening…..

Witness the sensations in your body. Be aware of what you are touching….

Know that you are watching yourself seeing, be aware of what you are looking at…..

Be aware of the flavour in your mouth, your sense of taste. Be aware of the act of eating, chewing, swallowing…

Be aware of your sense of smell, any odor or fragrance in the air, awareness of the breath flowing in and out of the nostrils…

Continue the state of *sakshi bhava* as long as you can while awake and while falling asleep. As you develop your ability to observe you are tuning into the intuitive aspect of your being.

## *Kayasthairyam* Body Steadiness

Develop stillness and steadiness of your physical body. Be the objective onlooker. Develop *sakshi bhava*, observing the external stillness of your body and the inner rhythmic movement of your breath. Eventually you will experience physical immobility as if you cannot freely move your body and yet your breath moves effortlessly. There is a dual awareness of the external stillness and the inner movement.

## *Yoga Nidra*™ Deep Relaxation

The Sanskrit term *yoga nidra*™ literally refers to "the divine sleep that occurs during dissolution". The modern technique of *yoga nidra*™ is the inspiration of Paramahansa Swami Satynanda Saraswati. At the onset of *yoga nidra*™ you mentally repeat a resolve about your goal. This resolve is known as *sankalpa*, a perfect thought process. When you make your *sankalpa* resolve avoid using the words no or not. For example, "From this moment I am….", or "I am….", "I feel….", "I know I am….". At first you may find it easier to imagine or visualize yourself achieving your goal rather than putting it into words.

When you practise *yoga nidra*™, as with any other yoga practice, unplug the phone, turn off your mobile phone and isolate yourself for the duration of the practice. Lie comfortably in *shavasana*. If your lower back is uncomfortable place rolled blankets under your knees. Use a thin cushion under your head so that the back of your head does not become tender during the practice. You may find it easier to record the practice. Speak slowly and allow pauses where indicated. Do not practise *yoga nidra*™ while driving your car!

Lie in *shavasana* and make all necessary adjustments so you can practise without distraction from your clothing, hair or blanket.

Develop the state of *sakshi bhava*. Be aware that part of your mind is standing back watching objectively. You are the silent onlooker of all the other aspects of your mind and body. Observe any mental chatter, let your thoughts go, be the witness of your personality, your intellect, your memories, your senses: smell, taste, sight, sensation, hearing. As experiences occur observe them, let them be, let them go and keep your awareness moving with the instructions.

During *yoga nidra*™ your extroverted mind will relax, the subconscious mind will surface. You may dream or have past memories that may be pleasant or unpleasant. Be the witness without involvement. Simply observe objectively.

Think of your *sankalpa* and repeat it mentally three times. Or visualize/imagine yourself working towards your goal and achieving it.

Now bring your awareness to your right hand and let go of all resistance in the right thumb, index finger, middle finger, ring finger, little finger, wrist relaxing, forearm, elbow, upper arm, arm pit, shoulder.

Keep your awareness moving, relaxing down the right side, chest muscles, waist, abdomen, hip, buttock, back of your thigh, top of the thigh, knee cap, back of your knee, calf muscle, ankle, heel, sole of your foot, ball of your foot, right big toe, second toe, third, fourth, little toe relaxing. Whole of the right side of your body relaxed.

Now move your awareness to your left hand. Relax your left hand thumb, index finger, middle finger, ring finger, little finger, wrist, forearm, elbow, upper arm, armpit, shoulder. Keep your awareness moving down the left side, relax your chest muscles, waist, abdomen, hip, buttock, back of your thigh, top of your thigh, knee cap, back of your knee, calf muscle, ankle, heel, sole of your foot, ball of your foot, left big toe, second toe, third, fourth, little toe. The whole left side of your body relaxed.

Right side, left side, both sides relaxed. And in the center of your body, your spinal column, axis of your body, relaxing each vertebrae from the base of your spine into your neck, the whole spinal column relaxed. Lower back muscles relaxing, middle of the back, upper back, between your shoulder blades, whole of your neck and throat, back of your head, top of your head, forehead, all the muscles of your skull. Right eyebrow, left eyebrow, eyebrow centre relaxed. Whole right eye, muscles around the eye, behind the eye. Whole left eye, muscles around the eye, behind the eye. Right temple left temple, right ear, left ear, the nose, nostrils, skin below the nose, upper lip, lower lip, gums, tongue from tip to root, whole of your mouth, lower jaw, the whole face, the whole head and whole external body, skin that covers your body, largest organ, relaxing.

Now internally your heart and lungs are moving rhythmically. Digestive system is relaxing, urinary, reproductive systems relaxing, whole nervous system and the skeletal system, inner structure of your bones relaxing… Every cell internally and externally relaxed.

Be aware of the space in front of your closed eyes. Your eyes are closed and you can still see. Look into that space and create an idea or an image. Imagine you are lying on green grass. Feel the earth beneath you. Imagine you are looking at the blue sky. You can see cloud formations, watch the shapes the clouds form…a dinosaur, a dragon, a horse, a house with a window, a flower, see what arises.

Now imagine you are encased in a bubble of rainbow coloured light. Let the light nurture you and protect you. Feel yourself floating in this bubble of light and see where the bubble carries you to.

Now come back to your physical body. Feel the stillness of your body and the movement of your breath. Know you are practising *yoga nidra*™. Remember your *sankalpa* and repeat it mentally three times or see yourself working towards your goal and achieving it.

Know that the practice of *yoga nidra*™ is drawing to a close. Have full awareness of your body. Slowly inhale feeling every part of your being, slowly exhale externalizing to the room in which you are lying and the surrounding environment. Gradually begin to move your fingers and toes. Swallow and then turn your

head from side to side. Stretch your arms above your head. In your own time roll to your side and sit. The practice of *yoga nidra*™ is now complete.

## *Soham Hamso* **Mantra Meditation**

**Stage one:**
Sit comfortably. Develop *kaya sthairyam* and *sakshi bhava*. Take your awareness inside your body. In place of your spinal column, imagine a long thin hollow tube running vertically from your tailbone up into the base of your skull. Slow your breathing and incorporate *ujjayi pranayama*. Imagine your breath is ascending through this spinal tube as you inhale and descending as you exhale. Practise this for a minute or longer.

**Stage two:**
As your breath ascends it produces the sound *so*. Mentally repeat the sound *soooooo* with inhalation. As exhalation descends it produces the sound *ham* (*hum*). Mentally repeat *hammmmmm* as you exhale. Practise this for a few minutes or longer.

**Stage three:**
Become aware of the change over when exhalation becomes inhalation. The sound of the breath will appear to be *sooooo hammmmm* pause. Practise this for a few minutes or longer.

**Stage four:**
Now become aware of the change over when inhalation becomes exhalation. The sound of the breath will appear to be

*hammmm soooo* pause. Practise this for a few minutes or longer.

**Stage five:**
Then become aware of both pauses after inhalation and exhalation. *Sooooo* pause *hammmmm* pause *sooooo* pause *hammmmm* pause. Practise this for a few minutes or longer.

**Stage six:**
Be aware of the sound of your breath without any pauses. Listen to *soooo hammmm soooo hammmm soooo hammmm soooo* until you can't be sure which comes first *so* or *ham* or *ham* then *so*. Practise this for a few minutes or longer.

**To complete the practice:**
After exhalation leave the sound of soham and be aware of the breath ascending and descending in the spinal passage. Continue this awareness for 30 seconds or so.

After exhalation become aware of the physical sound of your breath at the throat.

Relax *ujjayi* breathing. Be aware of the spontaneous breath. Look into the space of *chidakasha*, the space in front of the closed eyes. Be aware of what you see in that space.

Come back to your physical body. The practise of meditation is completed. Feel the stillness of your body, any discomfort. Slowly release your position.

**Practice Two:**
In the second practice of *soham* meditation you follow the same steps as above and extend your awareness of the spinal passage from the tailbone to the centre of the head.

**Practice Three:**
In the third practice of *soham* meditation you follow the same steps as above and extend your awareness of the spinal passage from the tailbone to the crown of the head.

### *Aum* **Chanting:**

Sound is a useful tool to captivate the mind and induce meditation. Traditionally the mantra *Aum* can be used by anyone and have a beneficial effect. The ancient sages described that the 'A' sound in *Aum* specifically influences the conscious mind, the "U" sound influences the subconscious mind and the 'M' sound influences the unconscious mind. The *Mandukyopanishad* scripture states that *the syllable Aum is the universe. Everything that exists in the past, present and future is Aum. And that which exists beyond the threefold division of time is verily the Aum syllable.* Therefore it is recommended to recite the *mantra Aum* either verbally or mentally to pacify the mind and emotions and eventually transcend the finite mind.

To chant *Aum* verbally, inhale slowly and produce the sound in a deep tone. When your mind is extroverted you tend to chant the A sound for a longer duration than the U or M sounds. As your mind starts introverting you will produce the M sound for a longer duration and the A sound will decrease in duration.

Sit comfortably. Develop *kaya sthairyam* and *sakshi bhava*. Inhale up from the earth through the spinal passage to the centre of the head and exhale out through the eyebrow centre while verbally chanting the sound of Aaaau-uuuummmmm. Practise for five minutes or so and then observe the space in front of your closed eyes and the feeling in your chest.

## *Tratakam* **Eyes Open Steady Gazing Meditation**

*Tratakam* gazing is practised with an object of choice, kept at eye level, one arm's distance from you. If you normally wear glasses and cannot see without them then continue wearing your glasses during the practice. If you can see without your glasses then do not wear them. It is important that the backdrop behind your image is plain, preferably white, so that no other images influence your vision.

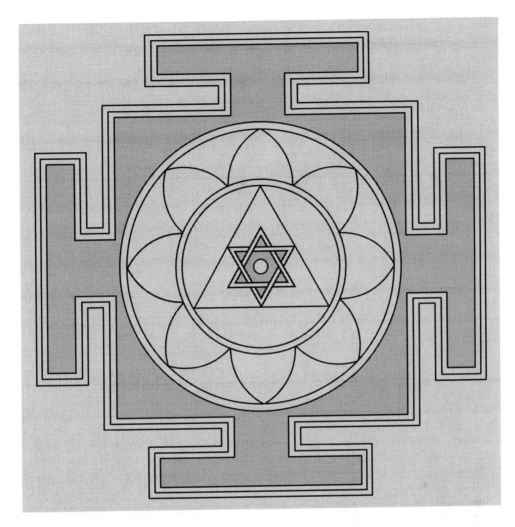

### Ganesha Yantra Tratakam:

A *yantra* is a specific geometrical form used in *tantra*. It is a vehicle for a particular form of universal energy. When you focus your gaze and mind on a *yantra*, it assists in awakening your own dormant energy and knowledge. The purpose of *Ganesha yantra* and *mantra* is to arouse stability and remove obstacles hindering your spiritual journey.

Sit comfortably. Develop *kaya sthairyam* and *sakshi bhava*. Gaze into the centre of the *yantra* form. Keep your eyes fixed at the central point. Repeat the *mantra* sound vibration of the yantra form: **Aum gam Ganapataye namaha**. *Mantra* can be practiced mentally or vocally. Check the pronunciation with the chart at the beginning of the book if you are unsure how to say the *mantra*. Keep in mind that Sanskrit is phonetic so sounds such as *gam* will be pronounced as gum.

While gazing at the *yantra* keep your eyes as steady as possible. If your eyelids are relaxed you won't need to blink often. Observe any thoughts that arise and keep your awareness on the *mantra* sound.

When you have finished, close your eyes, discontinue repeating the *mantra* and observe whatever you see with your eyes closed. Watch the image/s, color/s or patterns that arise and continue to observe your thoughts.

In the beginning practise for five minutes and gradually increase to 10 minutes.

## *Sphatika Tratakam*
**crystal gazing:**

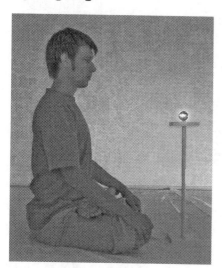

To practise crystal gazing, choose a clear quartz crystal stone or ball that appeals to you. If you are visual and have a psychic personality images will appear in the stone after 15 to 20 minutes of practice. Before practising you need to clear the energy that has previously collected in

the stone. Crystal emits electromagnetic energy and needs to be cleared periodically of any negative energy build up. To do this you may keep your crystal outside in the sunlight, moonlight, starlight, or soaked for 10 minutes in a saline solution containing a teaspoon or two of vinegar.

Hold your crystal in your left hand at heart level. Keep your right palm above your crystal without touching it. Close your eyes and mentally greet your crystal as a close friend. When you feel a sensation in your right palm then place your crystal on the stand. Sit comfortably. Develop the state of *kaya sthairyam* and *sakshi bhava*. Gaze into the centre of the crystal and keep watching with relaxed eyes and eyelids. Your eyes should not feel strained. Continue gazing without blinking often. Practise *chetana jagriti* while gazing.

When you have finished, close your eyes and observe whatever appears in front of your closed eyes. Watch the image/s, color/s or patterns that occur. Observe your thoughts.

## *Dipaprabha Tratakam*
**candle flame gazing:**

Sit comfortably and develop *kaya sthairyam* and *sakshi bhava*. Gaze into the centre of the flame and watch the shadowy area around the wick, not the flame itself. Look with relaxed eyes and eyelids, with as little blinking as possible. Your eyes should not feel strained. Keep your eyes focused. You may find you lose the image or have double vision, so adjust your vision when necessary. Close your eyes for a moment only if you have to. You should not strain your eyes in any way. Practise *chetana jagriti* while gazing.

When you have finished, close your eyes and observe whatever you see. Watch the image/s and or color/s that arise. Observe your thoughts.

## *Suryodaya Tratakam* **sunrise gazing:**

Stand or sit, outside if possible, while the sun is rising across the horizon. Practise *sakshi bhava*, gazing into the centre of the sun as long as it is a red or orange ball and repeat the sun mantra to focus your mind: **Aum ghrini Suryaya namaha.**

When you have finished close your eyes and observe whatever you see. Watch the image/s and or color/s that arise. Observe your thoughts.

This is a useful practice to prepare you for the coming day.

## *Suryastam Tratakam* **sunset gazing:**

The same practice can be done at sunset. It is a useful practice to prepare you for slowing down for the night.

## *Purnima Tratakam* **full moon gazing:**

Stand or sit, outside if possible, and gaze into the centre of the full moon. Practise *sakshi bhava* and repeat the moon mantra to keep your mind focused: **Aum Chandraya namaha** or **Aum soma Somaya namaha**. When you have finished close your eyes and observe the space behind your eyelids. Watch the image/s and or color/s that occur. Observe your thoughts.

## *Sphatika Shuddhi* **cleansing with crystals**

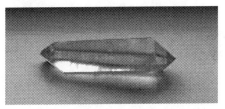

Find yourself four quartz crystals that have a termination at each end, called double terminated crystals. Your crystals should be cleaned first before using them. Either place them outside in the sunlight, moonlight or starlight for 12 hours or soak them for 10 minutes in a saline water with one or two teaspoons of vinegar and then rinse them under fresh water.

During the practice of *sphatika shuddhi* lie in *shavasana* and lay the crystals around your body with each termination pointing towards you. When you lie down one crystal should be placed below your feet; another two crystals either side of your hands and the fourth crystal above your head.

Develop *sakshi bhava*. Now imagine white light pouring in through the crystals and filling you with white light. Allow the light to clear all the debris from your body, mind and emotions.

When you feel clear and clean, give thanks for receiving the light. Leave the practice. Observe the space in front of your closed eyes until you are ready to get up. To enhance *sphatika shuddhi*, practise outside at sunrise.

## Timing your practice

To time your practice you can use a **mala** rosary rather than looking at the clock. By using a *mala* rosary you don't have to set an alarm clock and so it is less invasive. Also if you start to fall asleep you will drop your *mala* and that will wake you.

A *mala* has 108 beads made specifically of *tulsi* (ocimum sanctum) or sandalwood, crystal, coral and other semi precious stones, shell or *rudraksha* (elaeocarpus granites) seeds. Each time you repeat a *mantra* you move a bead. Between the 108th bead and the first bead is a **sumeru** tassel. When using a *mala* you do not move your fingers past the *sumeru*, instead you turn the *mala* around to start again.

To hold your *mala* you join your thumb and ring finger tips around the beads and let the *mala* hang down. Each time you repeat a *mantra*, move one bead with your middle finger. It may take 10 min-

utes to turn the 108 beads depending on the length of your *mantra*. If you do not wish to repeat a mantra you can turn a bead after each exhalation. Do a trial run first to find out how long it will take you to turn the whole *mala*. If it takes too long tie a piece of string after 54 beads and practise half a *mala*.

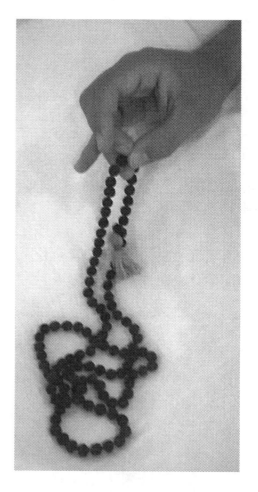

# CHAPTER NINE

# Food & Health Tips

*That which you see feeds your mind,*
*That which you hear feeds your heart,*
*That which you touch feeds your feelings,*
*That which you smell feeds your memory*
*And that which you taste feeds your body.*

(Muktibodha)

There is a lot of information today on specific foods to assist your health, so much so that it can be overwhelming. As you know, eating correctly is essential for a healthy body and mind. You need a balanced diet of fibre, protein, slow release carbohydrates and good fats, but what are your specific needs? While food is your means of survival, it also constitutes your chemical make up and influences the way you feel and think. If, for example, you have a thyroid deficiency then you need to avoid foods that come into the goitrogen category otherwise you will exacerbate the problem. If you are allergic to gluten then you need to avoid wheat, barley and rye. If you have a leaky gut then you need to eat foods that are low in amines. When you are going through peri menopause and menopause then you need phyto oestrogens. And so the list of food necessities and intolerances go on and on.

Yoga categorizes foods according to their influence on the body and mind. Foods that make you feel heavy and lethargic after eating are **tamasik** foods, such as alcohol, red meat or those lacking *prana*, which are stale or have been dehydrated, tinned or kept in the refrigerator for a long time. Food that heats your body and activates the reproductive glands is **rajasik,** such as hot peppers, chillies, black pepper, onions and garlic. Foods that harmonize and nourish the body, mind, emotions and spirit are **sattvik,** such as milk, yoghurt, ghee, fruits, vegetables, almonds and grains.

*Ayurvedic* medicine is very thorough in its definition of what you need to eat depending on the balance or imbalance of three **dosha** substances in your body. These *dosha* substances are known as **vata** air content and digestive gas, **pitta** bile and acidity, **kapha** mucous and phlegm. Every one is a combination of each *dosha*, though one or two may predominate. Listed below are the idiosyncrasies of these *dosha* substances and the appropriate foods for each. Although red meat is a good source of vitamins and minerals, according to *ayurveda*, consuming it tends to imbalance each *dosha* and is therefore not recommended. However, you may need red meat for specific reasons and should therefore balance it with other complementary foods.

## Symptoms of an imbalance of the *kapha* **phlegm** *dosha*:

- excessive mucous, blocked sinuses and hay fever
- cough, cold, flu, bronchitis, asthma, pneumonia
- sluggish digestion
- oily skin
- slow metabolism, gain weight easily, water retention
- endomorph body type with a tendency to gain weight

## Foods to avoid when *kapha* is over productive:

- cold or frozen food
- drinks from the refrigerator
- sweetened and sweet food, cane sugar, banana, avocado, coconut, dates, fresh figs, grapes, melons, oranges, papayas, pineapples, plums
- citrus fruit
- sour food, sour condiments and pickles
- salty food, seaweed, seafood, salty meats
- red meat and seafood
- dairy products

- castor oil, fried food and nuts
- wheat, oats, rice other than basmati, hot cereals, grains
- kidney beans, tofu
- flaxseed, sesame seeds, ginseng, psyllium

## Foods that balance *kapha* **mucous:**

- warm food
- buttermilk (not cold), yoghurt room temperature, diluted warm milk, *lass*i (not cold), small quantities of cottage cheese or *pani*r
- very small quantities of ghee, olive oil, corn oil, sunflower, safflower or almond oil
- small quantities of raw honey (not heated)
- spices and herbs such as pepper, basil, chamomile, cloves, cinnamon, echinacea, fenugreek, fennel seeds, coriander, cumin, dill, garlic, ginger, mace, parsley, peppermint, spearmint, nutmeg, sage, sweet curry leaf, turmeric, marjoram, mustard seeds, neem or margosa (azadirachta indica) leaves, oregano, paprika, pau d'arco, rosemary, St. John's Wort, tarragon, thyme
- cooked vegetables, artichoke, asparagus, broccoli, brussels sprouts, beetroots, cabbage, carrots, cauliflower, celery, daikon, eggplant, garlic, gotu kola (pennywort), green beans, green mustard leaf, leafy green vegetables, kohlrabi, kunkung, lettuce, okra, onions, peas, peppers, potatoes, radish, spinach, alfalfa, bitter tasting vegetables, such as bitter melon/gourd, kale, radishes
- apples (raw and cooked), apricots,

berries, cherries, cranberries, figs, mangoes, peaches, pears, cooked pears, prunes, pomegranates, dried fruits, in particular dried apricots, figs and raisins, very small quantities of lime zest
- amaranth, barley, buckwheat, corn, millet, quinoa, dry oats, rye, sago, very small quantities of basmati rice, wheat, amaranth and spelt
- all legumes except kidney beans cooked mung beans, lima beans, black beans, red and brown lentils, toor (arahar) dal
- poppy seeds, sunflower and pumpkin seeds
- small quantities of chicken, turkey, shrimp, warm eggs (not fried)
- small quantities of diced tofu cooked with spices
- very small quantities of olive oil or ghee
- Eat your main meal at midday.

## Symptoms of an imbalance of the *pitta* bile *dosha*:

- excessive acidity in the digestive tract, reflux, ulcers, diarrhoea
- skin rashes, pimples, boils, abscess, hemorrhoids
- hot flushes
- excessive perspiration
- bloodshot eyes, other than allergy-related
- high blood pressure
- anger, irritability, hot temper, tantrums
- balding, early greying
- mesomorph body type with a tendency to be physically overactive

## Foods to avoid when *pitta* bile is excessive:

- castor oil
- sour food (except lemon because it neutralizes *pitta*)
- honey and molasses
- buttermilk, cheese, egg yolk, sour cream, yoghurt
- salt, salty food, seaweed, seafood (excluding shrimp), salty meats
- hot spices, pepper, red chilli, bay leaf, basil, cardamom, cloves, fenugreek, nutmeg, sage, rosemary, turmeric, ginseng, mustard seeds, paprika, parsley, tarragon, thyme
- beetroot, carrots, eggplant, garlic, hot peppers, radishes, spinach, tomatoes
- sour and unripe fruit, apricots, bananas, berries, sour cherries, cranberries, grapefruit, papaya, peaches, persimmons
- red meat and seafood in general
- brown rice, corn, millet, rye
- flaxseed, sesame seeds, pumpkin seeds
- fried foods, nuts
- almond oil, corn oil, safflower oil, sesame oil
- lentils
- vinegar, pickles and sauces, salt, sour salad dressings, spicy condiments

## Foods that balance *pitta* bile:

- whole milk and soft mild cheese, cream, sweet yoghurt drink
- sweet food in general
- cool foods from the fridge and freezer
- sweet spices and herbs in small quantities, cardamom, cinnamon, coriander, cumin, curry leaves, dill, fennel, basil,

mint, chamomile, echinacea, mint, parsley, pau d'arco, peppermint, saffron, spearmint, St. John's Wort, sweet orange zest, turmeric, wild yam, neem

- sweet and bitter vegetables, such as kale, bitter melon, raw and cooked vegetables, alfalfa, artichoke, asparagus, broccoli, brussel sprouts, capsicum, cabbage, cauliflower, celery, corn, cucumber, gotukola (pennywort), green beans, green mustard leaf, leafy green vegetables, lettuce, mushrooms, okra, peas, potatoes, sprouts, squashes, sweet green peppers, sweet potatoes, zucchinis
- sweet and ripened fruits, apples which are astringent, avocado, cherries, coconut, figs, dark grapes, mangos, melon, oranges, pears, pineapple, plums, watermelon
- psyllium
- prunes, raisins, dates
- legumes, lima beans, chickpeas, mung beans,
- soya bean products, small quantity of tofu, red and brown lentils
- white rice, especially basmati rice, barley, wheat, oats, amaranth
- small quantities of chicken, turkey and shrimp
- coconut, pumpkin and sunflower seeds, soaked almonds
- olive oil, coconut oil, ghee, soya oil, sunflower oil, walnut oil

## Symptoms of an imbalance in the *vata air* dosha:

- intestinal gas, constipation
- irregular and light appetite, weight loss
- light sleep, insomnia, nightmares
- indecisive, nervous, unnecessary, excessive anxiety, fear, worry,
- forgetfulness
- muscular spasm and cramping, joint pain, backache, earache
- poor circulation, cold hands and/or feet
- dry eyes, dry and wispy hair, dry cracked skin
- receding gums
- ectomorph body type with a tendency to lose weight

## Foods to avoid when *vata* air is excessive:

- bitter foods such as bitter melon, kale mustard greens
- hot peppers, chillies, coriander seeds, cumin, fenugreek, parsley, pungent spices, saffron, turmeric, chamomile, echinacea, mint, pau d'arco, St. John's Wort, neem
- astringent food
- cold food from the refrigerator and freezer,
- red meat
- dried fruits and food such as potato or corn chips, biscuits, wafers, crackers
- raw vegetables, alfalfa
- unless the following vegetables are sautéed with oil they should be avoided: broccoli, brussel sprouts, cabbage, cauliflower, celery, cucumber, eggplant, leafy green vegetables, mushrooms, peas, peppers, potatoes, sprouts, tomatoes, zucchini
- unripe fruits especially bananas, apples,
- apples, cranberries, pears, pomegranates,
- legumes and lima beans
- barley, buckwheat, corn, dry oats, millet, rye

- caffeine, coffee, chocolate, tea, gurana, coca cola

**Foods that balance** *vata* **air:**

- milk, dairy products (not cold or frozen)
- sweet foods, honey, maple syrup, molasses
- allspice, anise, asafoetida, basil, bay leaf, use black pepper sparingly, caraway, cardamom, fresh coriander leaf, cinnamon, cloves, cumin, fennel, fenugreek, garlic, ginger, ginseng, juniper berries, liquorice root, mace, marjoram, mustard seeds, nutmeg, oregano, sage, marjoram, paprika, rosemary, tarragon, thyme, parsley
- flaxseed, psyllium, sesame seeds
- milk, dairy products (not cold or frozen)
- cooked vegetables, particularly artichoke, asparagus, beetroot, carrot, corn, gotukola (pennywort), green beans, okra, cooked onions, squashes, sweet potato, turnips, small quantities of sautéed leafy greens, wild yam
- sweet fruits, ripe bananas, cooked apples, apricots, avocados, berries, cherries, coconut, fresh figs, kiwi fruit, mangos, sweet melons, papaya, pineapple, peaches, plums, dates, prunes, sour fruits, stewed fruits.
- salt, salty foods, seaweed

- vinegar
- cooked moist oats (not dry), wheat, cooked rice, especially basmati rice
- small amounts of chicken, turkey, sea food in general, white fish, eggs
- small quantities of tofu
- nuts, especially almonds, walnuts, hazelnuts and cashew nuts, almonds can be soaked overnight to have for breakfast
- roasted sunflower and pumpkin seeds
- cooked chickpeas, mung beans, red lentils
- ghee and all oils, especially castor oil, olive oil and sesame oil, except: canola, corn, soya and safflower

**When you have specific health issues**

It is always best to consult your health care practitioner when you have specific health issues. Medical practitioners can be of great benefit but other modalities can also be of use to cure the problem. Naturopathy, homeopathy, acupuncture and *ayurveda* are time-tested approaches to health. A very accurate modern day system of health combines acupuncture and homeopathy through Mora* bio-electric diagnosis and therapy. While many health issues can be lessened or alleviated through sensible *yoga* practice you may need to incorporate other modalities.

*Mora Therapy is electro acupuncture using German diagnostic equipment (as developed by Mr. F. Morell) in combination with the principles of Chinese medicine and homeopathy. By testing the energy potential of 20 acupuncture points, the Mora practitioner is able to ascertain the state of the organs and systems (such as respiratory, lymphatic, digestive circulatory systems, etc.), that pertain to each meridian, With the use of the Mora machine allergens, bacteria and viruses can be detected; vitamin supplements, foods, water, etc. can be tested and individual homeopathic remedies are included in the treatment circuit.

## Here are a few other health tips:

Most importantly try to avoid chemical additives in food, cosmetics, sun creams and shampoos. Get out into nature as much as possible, breath fresh air and drink pure water. There are so many stresses in life, if you can avoid added chemical stresses half your problems will be solved!

**Acne:** Can be caused for many reasons- hormonal, digestive or emotional stress. An external application of carrot oil may help, but most important is to make sure you drink water and cut down on excessive oil and sugar intake. Practise *yoga asana* daily for at least half an hour, *pranayama, yoga nidra*™, *manipura chakra shuddhi* and *anahata chakra shuddhi*.

**Andropause or viropause:** Generally affects men between the ages of 40 to 55, though it may occur sooner or later when there are obvious physiological, hormonal, chemical and psychological changes. The most common symptoms are slower recovery from injuries and sickness, less physical endurance, weight gain, loss of or thinning of head hair, deterioration of eyesight, disturbed sleep, poor concentration and memory, irritability, indecisiveness, anxiety and fear, depression, loss of self confidence, purpose, direction and happiness, feeling lonely, reduced interest in sex and erection difficulty. Modern medical science can help with these symptoms, though you may prefer to use herbs, maca powder, homeopathy, acupuncture, creative expression, exercise outside, *yoga* plus meditation. Eat plenty of vegetables, fruit, legumes and reduce red meat and dairy. Read books about male menopause so you are informed on the subject. All the *yoga asana* listed in this book are beneficial, also practise *pranayama, bandha, yoga nidra*™ and meditation.

**Anxiety:** Correct diet, homeopathy, *yoga asana, pranayama, yoga nidra*™, meditation, aromatherapy and massage assist in alleviating all kinds of stress. Also your general outlook on your life situations can cause your stress levels to rise or lower.

**Asthma:** First consult your doctor or health care therapist before including any practices from this book. If suitable, your daily regime can incorporate *shashankasana, saral bhujangasana*, dynamic *asana* postures, *pranayama* breathing excluding the cooling breath and *yoga nidra*™.

**Breast tissue pain:** Can occur when you are premenstrual or peri menopausal. It may be alleviated by drinking cranberry juice or taking cranberry tablets.

**Chronic fatigue syndrome:** May be a symptom connected to other imbalances or problems. It is important to sort out the cause of the problem, though this can be time-consuming and expensive. Correct diet and gentle *yoga* plus meditation may assist you through the process.

**Cough with mucous:** If you have a productive cough, discontinue eating dairy products and check the cause of your cough with your health care practitioner. Drinking liquorice root tea or black coffee (not instant) may relieve your symptoms. Alternatively, you could try tea made from a small amount of fresh ginger, a piece of cinnamon quill, five crushed cardamom pods, two cloves, a few black pepper corns and a bay leaf. Boil the ingredients and then add tea leaves. Strain the tea and add honey to taste. Do not go out in the cold wind after drinking this tea. An *ayurvedic* tonic known as *dasa-moola-rishtham* may be obtained from Indian or Sri Lankan grocers or *ayurvedic* consultant. Sniffing warm saline water and or your own urine can assist in removing the mucous. Use aromatherapy in an oil burner with peppermint, spearmint, eucalyptus and/or orange or lemon oil. Don't lie on your back during *yoga nidra*™, lie on your side.

**Dry cough:** Have a check up with your health care practitioner to find out the cause of your dry cough. Liquorice root tea or black coffee (not instant) can sometimes relieve a dry persistent cough. You could also try the tea made from ginger and spices as mentioned for above. *Dasa-moola-rishtham* may be of assistance. When you practise *yoga nidra*™ lie on your side, rather than your back, so you do not aggravate your cough.

**Depression:** There are many factors and disorders that induce a state of mental depression. The cause may be physiological stemming from an imbalance of hormone secretions or vitamins; or a metabolic disorder; or an impaired liver; or an underactive thyroid; or an age-related hormonal change and low levels of testosterone, oestrogen, pregnenalone or growth hormone; or a tumor; or a neurological disorder; or even diet-related such as gluten or amine intolerance. Depression may be the result of a disease such as arthritis, bipolar, Crohn's, cancer, fibromyalgia, multiple sclerosis, lupus, a low level of hydrochloric acid in the stomach, sub-clinical Parkinson's disease or Alzheimer disease. So you really need to consult your health care practitioner to determine if the cause is physiological. Depression can also be circumstantial due to events in your life. While you may be able to change some of your circumstances, you will need to learn to manage yourself in the ones you cannot change. *Yoga* philosophy can assist your attitudes and *Hatha Yoga* can assist the physiological and energetic causes. Depending on the severity of depression, it may not be advisable to practise *yoga nidra*™ or meditation. Homeopathy may be useful for the physiological and psychological imbalances causing depression.

**Digestive disorders:** Consult your health care professional regarding the source of your digestive problem. Chamomile tea can be of assistance when you feel bloated in the abdomen. Forward and backward bending *yoga asana* postures can be useful depending on the problem. *Pranayama, yoga nidra*™ and meditation also improve the digestive system. Helicobacter pylori bacteria may reside in the stomach and digestive system for many years before symptoms are noticed.

It is a common cause of digestive upset and eventually leads to more invasive problems and referred pain. Medically it is diagnosed by a blood and breath test and then treated with strong antibiotics. Homeopathic medicine can be very useful to permanently eliminate the problem. Should it develop into an ulcer, *shitali* or *shitkari pranayama* can give some relief as well as *yoga nidra™*. No backward bending *yoga asana* postures or *uddiyana bandha* should be practised if you have an ulcer. *Vajrasana* is good for indigestion, especially when practised after eating.

**Flu:** Temporarily stop practising yoga when you have the flu. Bed rest is the best remedy. The tea mentioned above made from ginger and spices may assist. Do not resume *yoga* until you have recovered. Though there are many strains of flu, *dasa-moola-ristham* may relieve the symptoms or even prevent its onset.

**Eczema:** Applying your own urine, *amaroli,* to the affected area may be of assistance. Let it dry and wash with water only if there is an odor.

**Heart disease:** Correct diet and gentle *yoga asana, pranayama, yoga nidra™* plus meditation is important if you suffer heart disease. As a precaution if you have high blood pressure, do not bend forward to the extent that your head is lower than your heart even if you are on medication. Use a cushion under your head when lying down.

**Hernia:** You may need an operation for a hernia so speak to your doctor about this condition. Do not practise backward bending *yoga asana* postures.

**Immune system:** Make sure you eat foods rich in anti oxidants and practise *shashankasana, pranayama* and *yoga nidra™* daily to improve your immune system.

**Insomnia:** Drinking chamomile or valerian tea prior to going to bed can be useful to aid sleeping. A dose of *dasa-moola-ristham* before bed may also induce sleep. Practising *yoga nidra™* in bed may send you to sleep. If you wake during the night and can't get back to sleep try *shashankasana* in bed with your pillow under your forehead and your arms placed in a comfortable position. Count your breath backwards from 50 to one, breathing in 50, breathing out 50, breathing in 49 breathing out 49.....then lie on your right side so that your left nostril is uppermost and you will start to breath predominantly through your left nostril which is conducive for sleeping.

**Mature onset diabetes:** Spending a short period of time outside in the sunlight during the early morning or in the late afternoon is particularly beneficial if you have diabetes. Gymnema sylvestre is a time tested herbal tea that may assist in stabilizing high blood sugar levels. Eat a suitable diet avoiding processed foods and sugar. Exercise daily and practise forward bending *asana* postures. Invest in a blood sugar monitor to check your blood sugar levels daily. Homeopathy may help control blood sugar levels. If you cannot control your blood sugar naturally you will need to take tablets or insulin.

**Menstrual difficulties:** Consult your health care practitioner if you experience menstrual problems. Specific herbal remedies, homeopathic medicine and maca powder may be useful when dispensed by an experienced practitioner. Forward and backward bending *yoga asana* postures affect the reproductive area, however if you suffer from heavy bleeding avoid backward bending. *Pranayama* is important for the nervous system and yoga nidra™ enables the body and mind to relax.

**Mid life crisis:** If possible, stay in a suitable *Ashram* for a period of time if you are at the point of a mid life crisis. Otherwise spend a few weeks in nature, living simply without a television, radio, newspapers and magazines or talking on the telephone. Practise a regular routine of *asana, pranayama, mudra, bandha, yoga nidra*™ and meditation. When you live simply and get back to nature you can clear your mind and emotions and have a better sense of your direction in life.

**Pre and peri menopause:** Includes the 10 years prior to the cessation of your menses and two years after. Diet and specific herbs, maca powder, homeopathy, acupuncture and massage all play an important role to help you through this gradual change. Reading books on the subject also gives you a better

understanding of yourself. As you enter this new phase of life it is important to have creative expression and spend time in nature. Be sure to practise backward and forward bending *yoga asana* postures daily, as well as *asana* postures that assist in maintaining strength and flexibility, *pranayama, bandha, yoga nidra*™ and meditation.

**Pregnancy:** Consult your health care practitioner to determine if *yoga* will be suitable during your pregnancy. Practise *yoga asana* within your capacity but do not perform inverted poses. After 10 weeks avoid backward bending, lying on your tummy or flat on your back with your legs stretched out. *Pranayama* and meditation are very important during this time. Your doctor and health care professional can advise you about your dietary needs. Homeopathic remedies can be useful if you experience morning sickness, or continual nausea as the case may be!

**Prostate gland:** Consult your health care practitioner if you have a problem with urinating, if there is blood or semen in your urine and you experience lower back or pelvic pain. To maintain a healthy prostate gland avoid saturated fats and eat good oils such as cold pressed virgin olive oil, avocado oil and macadamia oil. Eat lean meat if you are not vegetarian and cook it on a low flame no higher than 200 degrees centigrade. Be sure to eat plenty of fruits and vegetables and also include lentils in your diet. Practise *saral bhujangasana* daily followed by forward bending.

**Thyroid gland:** Having a blood test may reveal if your thyroid is under or overactive. However, the interpretation of your blood test is based on statistics. Therefore, keep in mind that there can be an individual variation from the norm and interpretation requires insight too. Natural therapies may assist to alleviate your symptoms or you may need to take conventional allopathic medicine. Read books on the subject to become more informed.

Symptoms of an underactive gland vary from person to person. These include lethargy and tiredness, low libido, weight gain, poor digestion, slow metabolic rate, dry skin, constipation, body aching and foot pain, loss or thinning of head hair, poor memory and concentration, mixing up words and forgetting words, headaches, irritability, moodiness, depression or can't face work, nasal mucous, feeling cold and sensitive to cold, frequent miscarriage, fibroids, abnormal menstrual cycle, carpal tunnel syndrome, poor balance, dizziness, goitre, recurring infections (such as throat or bronchial), shoulder blade pain, anxiety and fearfulness, family history of thyroid imbalance. When you have hypothyroidism avoid eating foods that are goitregens such as broccoli, cabbage, cauliflower and almond as they suppress thyroid function. Practise *yoga asana* postures that compress and stretch your throat; *ujjayi pranayama; yoga nidra*™ and *vishuddhi chakra shuddhi*.

Symptoms of an overactive thyroid gland include restlessness, over activity, sleeplessness, weight loss, increased metabolic rate, bulging eyes, enlarged pulsating thyroid gland, profuse perspiring, muscular tremoring, an overly strong heart beat, accelerated pulse, shortened attention span, snap decisions, frenetic behavior and tiring easily. Practise gentle *yoga asana* postures, *ujjayi pranayama, yoga nidra*™ and *vishuddhi chakra shuddhi*.

**Warts:** Apply your own urine, *amaroli*, to the wart daily and eventually it will either fall off or disappear.

# CHAPTER 10

# Relationships & Family

*Mother is nurturer and the central sun.*
*Father and Children are the planets*
*revolving around her.*
*Should the sun waiver*
*then all balance is lost.*

(Muktibodha)

Understanding your own and other people's behavior can be difficult sometimes. First of all you need to know yourself intimately. There may be some aspects of yourself or someone close to you that you prefer to be in denial about. Meditation, reflection and uncritical self-analysis are all important processes towards understanding your inner make up and that of others.

As an adult you respond to your environment from past conditioning and your inherent nature. When you are able to see your negative conditioning and reactions, then you have taken the first step towards positive reconditioning. This first step of acknowledging your negative

tendencies is possibly the hardest. The second step is to gradually accept the negative tendencies. And the third step is to retrain your mind and emotions with suitable guidance.

People have different natures and so your path of reconstruction will be different to the next person. For example, maybe you are an alcoholic. Attending Alcoholics Anonymous has helped you; however, your neighbor found counselling and hypnotism to be of more benefit. Or when you gave up smoking cigarettes, you simply stopped but your brother needed nicotine patches and constant encouragement. Quite often homeopathic remedies can restore emotional balance but it may not work if the dosage is incorrect. Your path to happiness may not be the same as others but the underlying issues are similar.

In order to understand yourself first look at your source of self-esteem. Are you comfortable within yourself when you drive a cheap car or do you need an expensive one? Can you live in a modest house or do you need more style to appear important to other people? Can you wear simple clothes and still feel good about yourself or do you need designer labels for self-importance? Or do you feel embarrassed having expensive designer items because they are too good for you? If your self worth is dependant on these external things then you need to develop worthiness about your own good qualities.

Then take a look at the type of people you are attracted to. Do these people accept you for who you are? Or do you have to live up to their standards? Do they degrade you in any way mentally, emotionally or physically? Or do you feel better than them? Perhaps your father abandoned you as a child, so as an adult you are always attracted to men who ultimately desert you. Perhaps your mother was a closet alcoholic and you are still attracted to addictive personalities. Maybe you were abused physically or emotionally and so you continue to form relationships with someone who degrades you. As an adult you gravitate towards familiar childhood relationships. Once you can see your patterns, then

you have a choice to correct them whenever you are ready.

Life is about choices and poor choices are a bonus to your learning. But eventually you will have to stop making those poor choices. Making healthy choices means acknowledging the aspects of yourself you don't like. It may be difficult to accept your shadow side because you think in terms of what is good or bad, of what you like or dislike. Try looking at your shadow self as your infant child. Whether your infant is good or naughty you still love your child. A naughty child needs a lot of caring and attention and so does your shadow self. The more you ignore or shut it out the more it will want your attention. Give it the love and attention it deserves in order to fill it with light and happiness.

Even if you think you don't have a problem you can still learn a lot by reading books on self-esteem, addictive personalities, co-dependency and loving too much. By understanding human nature and witnessing yourself objectively, practising *yoga nidra*™, *pratyahara* and meditation, you can start to deal with the subconscious tendencies and clear out underlying negative patterns.

## SARRB guideline

When you have the right approach to life it is far easier to find happiness. The SARRB methodology is based on fundamental principles: strategies, appreciation, respect, responsibility and boundaries.

Depending on what you need to learn in your life, you will find yourself continually in similar situations, even though the circumstances or people are different, until you know how to handle yourself and achieve a positive outcome. Therefore, you need to develop constructive strategies. You may find counselling useful or talking to a friend beneficial or be able to devise your own strategies based on reading and introspection.

Sit quietly and look at the issue objectively before it occurs again and develop your strategy. For example, you may find it difficult to refuse when asked to do something, so you do it because it is easier than declining. Alternatively, you could say you will let the person know later. This will give you time to think about what you really want and how you are going to say it. Perhaps you are being bullied at work- you could try visualizing or imagining yourself encased in an egg of white light that is impervious to bullying and negativity. Maybe you live on your own and feel unsafe- have a plan of how you would ring the police and escape. To have a strategy means you are prepared rather than reacting impulsively. And as you live your life you will constantly find new strategies to deal with the situations that arise. The first strategy you can employ is to write your own understanding of each SARRB principle.

The next principle is to always appreciate. It is so easy to take things for granted. When you wake up in the morning what is the first thing you think of? Take a moment to appreciate the day, the small wonders and beauties of nature and the people around you as well as yourself and body. When you hug your child, parent, partner or friend, appreciate them for who they are and the joy or learning they give you. Through appreciation you will also develop the principle of respect.

Most importantly you need to respect yourself otherwise people will walk over you. When you can truly respect yourself you will find it easier to respect others as well as your environment. Nobody is perfect and if you develop respect then you will give yourself and others time to change.

So, by developing these principles you are taking responsibility for yourself and life. Each person has a role to play and a responsibility in that role. It is important to understand your responsibilities to others and yourself. This also includes emotional responsibilities, not just external duties. You have a responsibility to comprehend what others are telling; what your body is saying and what the earth is saying. You need to behave responsibly with others and yourself and to be generous of heart and spirit without being demolished. Even a child needs to know that as a family member they have to act accordingly. Everyone should be made aware of and think about his or her own responsibilities individually and collectively. When you acknowledge your responsibilities and those of others, you will create appropriate boundaries, which is the next principle.

While some people tend to be dominating and think that others should do and think the same as them, others find it easy to simply follow and be submissive. Perhaps you fit into both categories depending on the circumstance. Be aware of which category you fit into and utilise this pattern beneficially. Learn the appropriate action in any given situation and you will create a healthy boundary. If someone is abusive to you, you do not have to accept that abuse. Sometimes abuse is subtle and you do not see it at first. But once you recognize it, develop your strategy to handle the situation. If someone cannot take an initiative, offer constructive assistance without domination. It is essential to understand about boundaries for a healthy emotional life for yourself and others.

Living by the SARRB guideline will allow a smoother passage through your life. If your road still seems rocky do not be afraid to ask for help. Voice your issues to a friend, to the sky, even to yourself. It is possible to answer your own issues if you give yourself time and space.

## Family

The truth about healthy family dynamics is that the nurturer is the central pivot. It is up to the primary care giver to be strong, physically, mentally, emotionally and spiritually. Whoever plays the role of mother has centre stage and this needs to be fully understood. If the mother figure breaks down everything will fall apart even if the father is strong. If the father figure is weak while the mother figure is strong the family will still hold together.

Healthy dynamics start with being able to observe and witness. When you or your partner practise some form of introspective meditation you will have good groundwork for a healthy relationship. Not everyone is born with the ability to stand back and observe him or herself objectively. You have to work on it. The most valuable tool you can come into a relationship with is the ability to watch yourself objectively, to communicate and to listen. It is so important to be able to talk calmly about your feelings and needs and to ask your partner about his or her needs.

At the onset of your relationship discuss your goals. Before you even live together or get married find out what each other wants and expects in the relationship; where you hope to be in 10 years, 20 years, 30 years. Know that you are both on a similar path. Of course, hobbies and some interests will vary but your basic goals need to be the same and not opposing.

When you have issues, it is paramount to talk about these things. It is no use leaving your partner guessing. For example, it's your birthday and your partner forgets. So you get upset and sulk instead of saying, "today is my birthday". You become silent, brood and get angry about some other little thing that has no relevance. Then war breaks out and no one knows why! Understand yourself, your own dynamics and then understand the other person. Physiologically, men and women have different brains and process thoughts differently. If you and/ or your partner have difficulty expressing emotion then you need a safe environment and encouragement to express the emotion that is blocked. If you cannot resolve an issue between yourselves you may need a mediator. When you are caught emotionally in an issue you will need the help of an objective observer to bring clarity into the situation. Everyone has a conflict from time to time. That is how you grow. There is nothing to be embarrassed about asking for help. What is more important- your emotional sanity or keeping up appearances? By having healthy relationships with each other this reflects in your society as well as family and sends ripples around the world.

**Most important of all is to have fun. Enjoy your path to success as much as success itself.**

# Further Reading

There are many good books on the subject of *yoga* and spiritual life and abundant information on the Internet.

The books published by
**Bihar School of Yoga** and
**Sri Panchadashnam Paramahansa Alakh Bara**
are extremely informative. You can browse their website for a complete book catalogue and further information.
www.satyananda.net

*Kundalini in the Physical World*
by Mary Scott
Publisher: Routledge & Kegan Paul

*The Kundalini Experience*
by Lee Sannella MD
Publisher: Integral Publishing

*Theories of the Chakras: Startling insights into our energy system*
by Hiroshi Motoyama
Publisher: Lotus Press

*The Yoga of Herbs An Ayurvedic Guide to Herbal Medicine*
by Dr. David Frawley and
Dr. Vasant Lad
Publisher: New Age Books
www.motoyamainstitute.com/books.htm

*The Quick & Easy Ayurvedic Cookbook*
by Eileen Keavy Smith
Publishers: Journey Editions

*The New Glucose Revolution Achieve weight loss, blood glucose control and longlife health with GI*
by Prof. Jennie Brand-Miller,
Kaye Foster-Powell and
Prof Stephen Colagiuri
Publisher: Hodder Headline Australia P/L

*Eat Your Way Through The Menopause And Transform Your Life* and
*The New Natural Alternatives to HRT*
by Marilyn Glenville PhD
Publisher: Kylie Cathie Ltd

*The Hormone Connection How to Achieve a Better Hormone Balance: A Major resource for Every Woman*
by Gale Maleskey and
Mary Kittel
Publisher: Rodale

*Menopause The complete Australian guide to maintaining health, well-being and managing your life*
by Dr. Miriam Stoppard
Publisher: Dorling Kindersley P/L

# About the Author

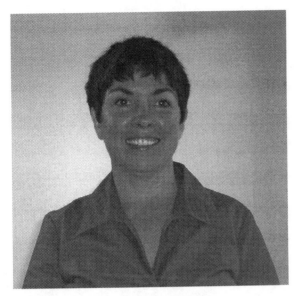

*Swami Muktibodhananda Saraswati*

Gabrielle Grace had an early calling to *yoga* at the age of 12 years. During her early childhood she was a student of classical ballet and later found greater fulfilment not only in the physical aspect of *yoga* but also in the philosophy and lifestyle.

In 1976 she met her mentor and *guru*, *Paramahansa Swami Satyananda Saraswati* whilst he was in Australia. She then travelled to India to study under his guidance for 10 years at Bihar School of Yoga, Munger.

Swami Satyananda initiated her into the *dasnami* order of *sannyasa* and she has since been known as Swami Muktibodhananda Saraswati.

During her time in India, Mukti authored and had published by Bihar School of Yoga, *Swara Yoga the Tantric Science of Brain Breathing* and *Commentaries on Hatha Yoga Pradipika, the Light on Hatha Yoga.*

In 1993 she received the title *Yogacharya, yoga* authority. Mukti has dedicated her life to the teaching and practice of all aspects of *yoga*.

Currently she teaches small groups, private classes and conducts seminars and integrates her yogic knowledge with family life.

Mukti can be contacted at muktibodha@yahoo.com.au

Printed in the United States
By Bookmasters